Biotechnologies and Reproductive Agency

As artificial reproductive technologies become available to populations that have previously not had access to them, this book asks how reproduction is being transformed by technologies and individuals whose sexual and reproductive lives may defy sociocultural norms, religious codes, and national laws.

Seeking to develop a novel approach for studying the families of the 21st century, it examines the uptake of assisted reproductive technologies (ART) by women who opt for solo motherhood, exploring the circulation of reproductive technologies, bodily material, and ideas in two countries recognized as leaders in ART and sexual and reproductive health rights. Through ethnographic research in Spain and the United Kingdom, it considers the ways in which the sociocultural, politico-legal, economic, and ideological intersections between solo-mother families and ART shape the experiences of those who take them up.

A multi-sited ethnography that explores the implementation, use, and experience of ART, this volume will appeal to scholars in the field of social sciences, human reproduction, science, technology and society (STS), policy studies, and people who are thinking about or have started a family with the help of ART.

Ana Bravo-Moreno is the Principal Investigator of an ERC advanced grant at the National Research Council (CSIC) in Madrid, Spain, and a tenured professor in social anthropology. She has been a research fellow at the IoE-University College of London (UCL), at the Institute of Migration Studies, Comillas University in Madrid, and at the University of Granada. She received her Ph.D. from the University of London that was funded by the Economic & Social Research Council, UK; she also holds an M.Sc. degree in Social Anthropology (UCL), and was an Erasmus student of M.A. in Women's Studies, Institute of Education, London, and has a B.A. (Hons.) in Philosophy at the Autonomous University in Madrid. She has been a visiting scholar at the University of California Irvine, UC-Berkeley, Brown University, and Florida International University. Her research has focused on assisted reproductive technologies, new family forms, reproductive health, international migration, and education.

Biotechnologies and Reproductive Agency

An Ethnography of Solo Motherhood in Spain and the United Kingdom

Ana Bravo-Moreno

Routledge
Taylor & Francis Group
LONDON AND NEW YORK

First published 2025
by Routledge
4 Park Square, Milton Park, Abingdon, Oxon OX14 4RN

and by Routledge
605 Third Avenue, New York, NY 10158

Routledge is an imprint of the Taylor & Francis Group, an informa business

British Library Cataloguing-in-Publication Data
A catalogue record for this book is available from the British Library

ISBN: 9781032209821 (hbk)
ISBN: 9781032217246 (pbk)
ISBN: 9781003269755 (ebk)

DOI: 10.4324/9781003269755

Typeset in Times New Roman
by Newgen Publishing UK

I would like to dedicate this book to my daughter, thanks to you I learned what unconditional love is.

Contents

Figure

Table

Preface

Aims of this book

This book is based on ethnographic research conducted in Spain and in the United Kingdom. It provides an analysis of the journey of choosing to become a solo mother through assisted reproductive technology (ART). It covers topics such as the decision-making process, interactions with healthcare professionals and fertility clinics, the fertility business, public policies regarding access to reproductive technology, balancing work and personal life, early childhood education, childcare, and children's schooling.

The objectives of this book are anchored in three thematic axes; in the first one I will examine solo motherhood by choice with the help of ART as experience: how personal stories and social histories intersect to enable women to pursue solo motherhood by choice; what are mothers' own perspectives on motherhood and mothering?; how these perspectives vary cross-nationally? Female-defined and female-centered experience of mothering is concerned with the meanings women attach to it. While the development of a feminist practice of gender socialization focuses upon the mother's relationship with her children and, in particular, the manner in which she raises them, hegemonic ideals of motherhood may be a site of oppression. Nonetheless, women's own experiences of mothering can be a source of power. The theory (O'Reilly, 2021; 2006; Rich, 1995) and practice of empowered mothering recognizes that both mothers and children benefit when the mother lives her life, and practices mothering, from a position of agency, authority, and autonomy. Therefore, this new perspective examines how mothers seek to imagine and implement a theory and practice of mothering that is empowering to women as opposed to oppressive. However, the emphasis on experience and empowerment from the perspective of individual women needs to engage with politics, economics, policy, and power. Therefore, truly to comprehend the complexities of such terms we need to broaden our awareness and understanding of the diverse positions and meanings of mothering without partners which is not a monolithic entity.

The second thematic axis has to do with motherhood as institution: how is that power exercised through specific social institutions and cultural ideologies?; how is motherhood enacted in and reinforced by public policy?; and how women juggle earning a living and parenting their children? Feminist historians (Knott & Taylor, 2005) agree that motherhood is not fundamentally a biological function but is primordially a cultural practice that is continuously being shaped in response to social and economic changes. As a cultural construction, its meanings vary over time and place; there is no essential or universal experience of motherhood. The current gender system and the socioeconomic structures in which we operate are not at all static. These values are not natural or neutral but are the reflection of a set of social, political, and economic interests that shape and constrain individual options. Some authors (Chodorow, 1978; Ginsburg & Rapp, 1995; Hochschild, 1989; Rich, 1995) reveal the ways in which women's choices in the family interact with unjust social structures outside of the family, specifically with segregated division in work or in the economy. Childcare is a highly time-consuming activity, and those people – mostly women – who raise children alone face far greater difficulties in pursuing a demanding professional career. Thus, the structures of work and family form a cycle of vulnerability that conditions their lives and opportunities. Feminist scholars (Adkins, 1995; Allen, Walker, & McCann, 2013; Okin, 1989) indicate the way in which families are part of a system of social structures and cultural expectations that reproduces the social and economic inequality of women.

Families cannot be viewed apart from that system or in isolation from it. Furthermore, a choice by parents to participate in a gendered family affects the lives of their children. The free choices of such parents generate unequal opportunities for their children, inequalities that children themselves have not chosen. Standpoint theorists (Haraway, 1991; Harding, 1991, 2004, 2009; Hill Collins, 2004; Hooks, 1994; Wylie, 2017) argue that experiences of the marginalized reveal problems to be explained; problems that can become research agendas or policy issues and are a source of objectivity-maximizing questions. Thus, social-scientific research should "start out from" the lives of unprivileged groups in order to gain more knowledge of social reality. They suggest that research that begins from the lives of unprivileged groups enables social scientists to reveal "hidden aspects of social relations between genders and the institutions that support these relations" (Harding, 1991, p. 127). Implicit in Harding's suggestion is the argument that relations of power pose a special challenge for the methodology of the social sciences because they include "hidden aspects". Such questions force us to examine the beliefs, prejudices, and biases of the dominant groups in society, the propositions that have previously counted as knowledge. It is in this way that this book proposes we achieve less partial and distorted understandings of the lives of solo mothers by choice with the help of ART than if we allow questions about those lives to originate only from the experiences of dominant groups. The realities of these women's lives, then, can provide sites of enquiry that lead to new, more complete knowledge.

Finally in the third thematic axis, I will explore solo motherhood by choice and reproductive technologies as site for social change: how do women manage the gender hierarchy of daily life which they cannot control while they may simultaneously encourage their children to resist it? And do women who consciously choose solo motherhood challenge traditional practices of gender socialization for their children? According to Hertz (2006) solo mothers by choice speak of wanting their daughters to have positive images of female power and to see women as capable, having careers, and raising a family, they present a model of women as free to make choices they deem necessary for their own well-being, while successfully coping with pressures those choices entail. At the same time, they may want their sons to express themselves as individual people, acknowledging gender as only one of many components of their identity. Women may experience the tension between the freedom that they hope to provide for their children and the role models that they perceive they must provide, the tension between ideology and practice.

This study contributes to the field of social sciences and biotechnology in four important ways: (1) it will examine three interconnected aspects of motherhood: motherhood as institution, solo motherhood by choice with the help of ART as experience, and as a site for social change. This research investigates what changes are needed in social policy, education, the workplace, and the family to improve gender equality for mothers. (2) It aims to provide an understanding of the complexities of politics, culture, economics, policy, and power from an interdisciplinary perspective in order to broaden our awareness and understanding of the diverse positions and meanings of motherhood with the help of ART. (3) This work aims to construct a more complex understanding of the ways in which discourses of maternity shape and are shaped by various practices and experiences cross-nationally; and (4) it will illuminate how families may be a site of empowerment and a location of social change for women who resist replicating "conventional" forms of motherhood and raising children who may or may not conform with gendered expectations.

References

Adkins, L. (1995). *Gendered work. Sexuality, family and the labour market.* Open University Press.

Allen, K. R., Walker, A. J., & McCann, B. R. (2013). *Handbook of marriage and the family.* Springer.

Chodorow, N. (1978). Mothering, object-relations, and the female oedipal configuration. *Feminist Studies*, *4*(1), 137–158. https://doi.org/10.2307/3177630

Ginsburg, F., & Rapp, R. (Eds.) (1995). *Conceiving the new world order: The global politics of reproduction.* Berkeley, CA: University of California Press.

Haraway, D. J. (1991). *Simians, cyborgs, and women: The reinvention of nature.* London: Free Association Books.

Harding, S. (1991). *Whose science? Whose knowledge? Thinking from women's lives.* Ithaca, NY: Cornell University Press.

Harding, S. (Ed.). (2004). *The feminist standpoint theory reader. Intellectual & political controversies.* New York: Routledge.

Harding, S. (2009). Standpoint theories: Productively controversial. *Hypatia*, *24*(4), 192–200.

Hertz, R. (2006). *Singles by chance, mothers by choice.* New York: Oxford University Press.

Hill Collins, P. (2004). Learning from the outsider within: The sociological significance of black feminist thought. In Sandra G. Harding (Ed.), *The feminist standpoint theory reader: Intellectual and political controversies* (pp. 103–126). New York: Routledge.

Hochschild, A. R. (1989). *The second shift: Working parents and the revolution at home*. New York: Viking.
Hooks, B. (1994). *Teaching to transgress: education as the practice of freedom*. London: Routledge.
Knott, S., & Taylor, B. (Eds.) (2005). *Women, gender and enlightenment*. New York: Springer.
Okin, S. M. (1989). Reason and feeling in thinking about justice. *Ethics*, *99*(2), 229–249.
O'Reilly, A. (2006). *Rocking the cradle; thoughts on motherhood, feminism and the possibility of empowered mothering*. Toronto: Demeter Press.
O'Reilly, A. (2021). *Matricentric feminism: Theory, activism, practice*. Toronto: Demeter Press.
Rich, A. (1995). *Of woman born: Motherhood as experience and institution*. New York: W. W. Norton & Company.
Wylie, A. (2017). What knowers know well: Standpoint theory and the formation of gender archaeology. *Scientiae Studia*, *15*(1), 13–38.

Acknowledgments

Thanks to my mother who helped me take care of my daughter for a few weeks when I had to dedicate more time to finish off writing the research proposal to obtain funding for this project, just as my grandmother took care of me when my parents worked.

Thanks to all the participants who generously shared their own experiences with me.

Thanks to the European Commission for providing funding under the Marie S. Curie (H2020) Grant (number 797880), I was able to conduct this study. And thanks for the funding from the European Research Council Grant (number 101097431), I can continue with my current research project that allows me to study new family forms and assisted reproductive technologies today.

Earlier versions of some chapters were previously published in:

Chapter 1: Bravo-Moreno, A. (2017). Politics, doctors, assisted reproductive technologies & religion: Transgenerational understandings and experiences of single motherhood in Spain. *Health Care for Women International, 38*(10), 1058–1074.

Chapter 2: Bravo-Moreno, A. (2019). Deconstructing "single" mothers by choice: Transcending blood, genes, and the biological nuclear family? *Sage Open, 9*(4).

Chapter 4: Bravo-Moreno, A. (2022). Reproductive agency, assisted reproductive technology & obstetric violence. *Health Care for Women International, 43*(7–8), 806–826.

Chapter 5: Bravo-Moreno A. (2021). The intersection of reproductive, work–life balance and early-education and care policies: 'Solo' mothers by choice in the UK and Spain. *Social Sciences, 10*(12), 458.

Chapter 6: Bravo-Moreno, A. (2019). Choice mums and children's education. Does feminism matter? A qualitative study. *The Qualitative Report, 24*(4), 921–947.

Introduction

Solo motherhood is on the rise everywhere in the world. A Pew Research Center study of 130 countries and territories shows that the United States has one of the world's highest rate of children living in single-mother households (Kramer, 2019). Single parents now constitute about 19% of the households with children in the European Union. In the overwhelming majority of cases, this phenomenon concerns women. Only 15% of single parents are fathers, and their socioeconomic condition is better than that of single mothers. Not only are single mothers on the rise, but their situation is in many ways more challenging than that of other women. Indeed, single mothers are more likely to fall into poverty (their risk of poverty is 30% compared with 17% for couples with children), to have taken a part-time job in order to combine professional and family life, and to suffer poorer physical and mental health (Heine, 2016). The newest type of single-mother family comprises solo heterosexual women who have chosen to parent alone and adopt or have had children through assisted reproductive technologies (ART), the most common forms of fertility treatments are in vitro fertilization (IVF), intracytoplasmic sperm injection (ICSI), sperm donation, egg donation, embryo donation, and surrogacy. These women are generally referred to as "single mothers by choice". Exact figures, are yet to be provided for this type of family formation, even in countries with detailed records on ART treatments (European Society of Human Reproduction and Embriology, 2017). The number of single-mother-by-choice families has risen sharply since the millennium and is likely to grow given the demographic shift towards older first-time motherhood. Indeed, a significant proportion of those who now seek fertility treatment are women without a male partner. According to HFEA (2015) there was a 226% increase since 2006 in the United Kingdom, and in Spain the number increased fourfold in the last seven years. Studies have shown that single mothers by choice are generally well-educated women in professional occupations who become mothers in their late thirties or early forties. Children of single mothers by choice, however, have not been exposed to parental conflict and are less likely to experience the financial difficulties or maternal psychological issues that often occur as a consequence of marital breakdown or unplanned single motherhood (Jadva et al., 2009).

DOI: 10.4324/9781003269755-1

Selection of cases

Spain and the United Kingdom are two leading countries in ART and they are also two of the most advanced in sexual and reproductive health rights. Both countries (1) have legislation governing ART, whether independently or as part of broader legislative frameworks; (2) supplement legislation with professional guidelines; (3) are in the top 23 country league table of the world's best national health systems (CeoWorld, 2021); while (4) neither country discriminates against individuals for their sexuality or marital status, although access to gestational surrogacy is prohibited. Nevertheless, the laws in these two countries are not internally consistent. This has three consequences: (1) permissive legislation on one issue of regulation, for example, solo women or lesbian couples, does not guarantee access to ART for all solo women or lesbian couples; (2) differences in regulations indicate complex contradictions at national level and bureaucratic obstacles to legal parenthood; and (3) affordability affects access to ART treatment in these countries (Crawford et al., 2016). According to the data presented by ESHRE (2021), Spain constitutes 40% of the ART procedures carried out in the whole of Europe. Many factors contribute to the large influx of international patients to Spain seeking a chance to become a parent. Some of these include: (1) lower-cost treatment; (2) flexible laws: except for surrogacy, a patient is eligible for all types of reproductive procedures; (3) a reliable healthcare system; (4) leading fertility professionals; and (5) high success rates. Additionally, the country has a pool of anonymous egg and sperm donors at hand, helping patients to have a greater chance at a successful pregnancy. This is in contrast to the United Kingdom, where in 2005 the legislation was changed, requiring any donor of gametes or embryos used in the treatment of others to agree to the disclosure of their identity to any offspring reaching the age of 18 years. This caused a shortage of donors to which the participants in the United Kingdom allude, forcing them to resort to sperm banks abroad, such as Denmark and the United States, as well as egg donors, mainly in Spain.

Theoretical approach and research methodology

This study employs a feminist-standpoint approach (Haraway, 1991; Yuval-Davis, 2015; Wylie, 2017) that makes two principal claims: (1) knowledge is socially situated; (2) research aims to study the terms and understandings of the target groups to give an in-depth insight into the particular settings where the participants' ideas on ART, motherhood, mothering, and their children's education have been formed and conditioned by multiple factors. Haraway (1991) argues that (bio)technologies ought to be analyzed as situated practices that are unfolding expressing the entanglement of science, theory, and politics. The epistemology and methodology are rooted in the idea that three levels of analysis should be considered: sociocultural, institutional, and experiential. This approach structures and limits the comparative research design, focusing upon diverse national policy issues, political developments in Spain and the United Kingdom, and the transnational fertility care industry.

The use of a comparative cross-national approach allows for a more detailed analysis and a more comprehensive comparison when studying a smaller number of countries. This approach also facilitates consistency in defining and applying concepts, as well as using qualitative evidence. Qualitative approaches enable the investigation of the range of factors that can affect overall outcomes and provide detailed exploration of those that underpin participants' experiences of policy programs (Purdon et al., 2001). This is certainly a necessary requirement to achieve a broader, multidimensional approach for cross-national comparison. Using qualitative ethnographic methods from a standpoint approach will make visible aspects of social relations that are unavailable from hegemonic perspectives, and in so doing they generate the kinds of questions that will lead to a more complete account of those relations. In addition, this data can form rich sites for research, for policy reform and, ultimately, for social change.

This study draws on ethnographic research that took place in London (the United Kingdom), Madrid and Andalusia (Spain), where I carried out a total of 70 interviews: 60 in-depth interviews with solo mothers by choice who used ART, 30 in London and 30 in Madrid and Andalusia will constitute the main part of the sample. Participants in this study were chosen through the snowball method which began among different groups of acquaintances and associations of solo mothers by choice. They were diverse in age, ethnicity, sexual orientation, class, and education level, number of children and their children's age. Purposive sampling was used to ensure that a broad range of such mothers were recruited. The request for participants was distributed through associations, relevant internet websites, professional and leisure networks, as well as snowballing. In addition, ten semi-structured interviews were conducted in Spain and in the United Kingdom with NGOs and charities that dealt with donor-conceived families.

Prior to the commencement of this study and under the auspices of my university, I was required to gain ethical approval to ensure that this research conformed with general ethical principles and standards. The aim of the ethical review was to protect participants as a valuable part of the research process and not merely a means of accessing data as well as protecting the researcher. All participants freely provided their informed consent, ensuring that confidentiality and anonymity were strictly maintained, and data was securely handled. In-depth interviews were conducted at the women's homes, workplaces, cafeterias, and parks. They lasted on average two hours and were tape-recorded, and I met with some of these women for a second interview as they had other obligations and could not spend more time on our first interview. Interviews were organized around several topics: the decision to become a solo mother with the help of ART, the women's family of origin, support networks, mothering, work–life balance, public policies, feminism, and their children's education. I used an interview guide, and after several interviews the questions were flowing. I designed open questions that participants could understand and interpret in the way in which they were intended, taking into account terminology, avoiding jargon and ambiguous words, or words that could be misinterpreted. Questions were worded in a balanced way to guard against response bias, taking also into account that some women were caught between their "political correctness" and their antipathy to feminism, for example. As a whole, the questions were grouped into topics in a logical sequence to flow easily.

I use ethnography to construct a holistic understanding of the complexities of politics, policy, and power from an interdisciplinary perspective. Ethnography is based on the assumptions of understanding and interpretation of social events being processual, within the framework of naturalism and holism (Attia & Edge, 2017; Behar & Gordon, 1995; Hesse-Bibber & Piatelli, 2012; LeCompte & Goetz, 1982). As Sherry Ortner (2006, p. 42) argues, ethnography in its minimal definition is "the attempt to understand another life world using the self – as much of it as possible – as the instrument of knowing". The data analysis is based on grounded theory which helps the researcher using the empirical data to generate concepts and theories, moving through a process of discovery allowing the researcher to derive meaning from the data and analysis using creative, inductive processes (Taylor & Bogdan, 1998). Grounded theory also assists the ethnographer in maintaining control over the research process in focusing, structuring, and organizing it as this analytical method sustains a flexible approach to analyzing the empirical data and adds rigor to ethnographic research "by building systematic checks into both data collection and analysis" (Charmaz & Mitchell, 2007, p. 162), arriving at an understanding of a particular phenomenon from the perspectives of those experiencing it. All audio recordings were transcribed verbatim. Once all of the research interviews were transcribed, I began thematic analysis, approaching the data inductively, whereby theme development was directed by the content of the data: identifying issues, similarities, and differences, which were revealed through the interpretation of the participants' narratives. I was vigilant about my own experience and perspective, engaging in a self-reflective process where I put aside my own assumptions and experiential knowledge and paying attention to the participants' accounts with a broad mind.

I conducted the interviews between January 2017 and 2021, 30 of which were with women in Spain, between the ages of 36 and 57 years, who were heterosexual, university educated, middle class, and white. The other 30 in-depth interviews took place in London, between September 2018 and 2021 (Table A.1, Appendix). Most of these women stated that they were heterosexuals, with one bisexual and another pansexual, university educated, and between the ages of 35 and 65 years. In London, 17 participants are white British, 1 is a white South African, and 12 are white from European countries (Belgium, France, Ireland, Italy, Greece, Norway, Poland, Spain, Sweden, and Ukraine) who emigrated to London years ago.

The children of these women are between the ages of 5 weeks and 23 years, and were conceived through sperm donation and in 21 cases also with egg donation, with 4 cases of embryo donation. As a result of my fieldwork, I became a member of two associations: Madres Solteras por Elección (MSPE) (Single Mothers by Choice) in Spain, and the Donor Conceived Network (DCN) in the United Kingdom. I attended meetings, workshops, and conferences both in Madrid and in London from 2018, and also participated in the WhatsApp groups of both associations.

The ethnographic analysis incorporates a process of reflexivity that exposes all phases of the research activity to the continuous questioning and re-evaluation of the researcher. In keeping with standpoint theory, I am drawing reflexively on my own position to inform the data analysis (Collins and Gallinat, 2010; Ellingson and Ellis, 2008; Hancock, 2009).

Auto-ethnography

I have conducted this ethnography from my position as a woman who became a mother on my own by choice using ART in Spain, by far Europe's most active country in this technology (European Society of Human Reproduction and Embryology [ESHRE], 2017) and third in the world after the United States and Japan (FecunMed, 2019). Thus, I also take an auto-ethnographic approach as I became a mother with anonymous genetic material at a private clinic in Spain, and gave birth in a public hospital in 2011 in Spain. In this sense, I am able to draw directly from my experience and to contribute an insider perspective to observation and participation that are dependent upon the ethnographer's self. This experience has enabled me to immerse myself bodily and experientially as a technique of observation and analysis (Wacquant, 2004). Furthermore, Hancock argues that:

> While ethnography must be theoretically driven, it also must prioritize the elucidation of the practical knowledge of agents. This is premised on deep immersion utilizing the body as a vector of knowledge, is a methodological and theoretical tool to analyze the hidden material and symbolic dimensions that define a particular social world and the mutual penetration of agent and world.
>
> (2009, p. 94)

Similarly, Collins and Gallinat (2010, p. 17) explain that anthropologists should incorporate personal experiences as data in their analysis: "no anthropologist can afford to omit consideration of the possibility that they may themselves be their own, intimate informants". I lived in London (UK) for a total of more than 16 years and in Madrid and Andalusia (Spain) for more than 2 decades, and worked most of my adult life in both countries. My daughter was born in 2011, for the first seven years of my own daughter's life I lived in Spain, before moving to London for two years. In both places, I enrolled my daughter in a state school in the urban center. I participated in the educational communities of each school both as a mother and as an ethnographer. I was taking her to kindergarten and picking her up and going to the park. Participant observation was undertaken in parks where mothers, for the most part, and their children, aged between one and eight years, would gather, as well as my participation in parent meetings and children's parties over a nine-year period (2012–2021). I also kept a research diary and field notes of my interviews and observations made in different contexts: parks, schools, children's parties, and outdoor excursions as well as public events organized by fertility clinics in London and in Madrid. Throughout, I have tried to square the circle of being a mother and a worker without having a family or social network in any of the cities where I found myself, faced with policies of reproduction, work–life balance, and early-childhood education.

Hence this book is grounded in original empirical research and through an ethnographic lens attempts to understand the subject of study analyzing the legal, political, historical, economic, and sociocultural context. The aim is to rise above ideographic particularities to address wider theoretical questions. Although being a full member of the group under study means that one does not have a non-problematic position within that sample, the auto-ethnographer is more analytical and self-aware in the conversation of what it means to be a typical member of a group, being able at times to adopt an abstract or introspective standpoint of the conversation and the activities. The auto-ethnographer's understanding as a member of the group emerges not from detached discovery but from involved dialogue. Not only do auto-ethnographers form part of the representational process but they are also in part formed by those processes, given that the cultural meanings that they co-create are constituted in conversation, action, and text. The members of a group rarely show a uniform set of beliefs, values, and levels of commitment. Consequently, even the full member of a group gives only a partial viewpoint of the social world being examined. A central characteristic of this text is that the researcher is a highly visible element. The experiences of the researcher herself are incorporated in the story and are considered as essential data to understanding the social world under observation. Davies and Spencer (2010) underline that we should not lose sight of the ethnographic imperative, to understand and make sense of complex social worlds of which we only form a part. The ethnographic imperative demands a dialogue with the data or with other subjects and should be seen in terms of interrelations between researcher and the rest in order to inform about and change social knowledge.

Cultures, minds, and brains: experiences that enact and embody theory

My experience as a solo mother by choice with the help of ART connotes not just observation but also involvement and interaction in the social world as well as my own engagement with it. It is against this background that a phenomenological approach, based on the concept of experience, is key and this is why learning, anchored in the lived-body, is a central dimension of perception. Kondo (1990) argues that "the specificity of experience is not opposed to theory; it *enacts* and *embodies* theory". The concept of lived experience (Husserl, 1990), which is the focal point of phenomenology, suggests that consciousness and understanding cannot exist without being rooted in embodiment. The word Lebenswelt, introduced by Husserl (1990, p. viii), refers to the study of the world as it is subjectively perceived, rather than as an objective entity separate from the subject: "A living organism enacts the world it lives in; its effective, embodied action in the world actually constitutes its perception and thereby grounds its cognition".

The enaction paradigm provides a promising effort to offer a comprehensive understanding of cognition from the cellular level to society. It also embraces the necessity of exchanging information between individual subjective experiences and scientific methods as a fundamental approach. Contrary to previous theories that claimed that once brain architecture is created, it remains static, like computer hardware, is the recognition of the critical roles that brain plasticity plays in structure and function throughout life (Merzenich et al., 2013). Basic processes like learning and memory are facilitated by modifications in the connections and structure of neurons, such as the creation, fortification, and pruning of synapses (Cirelli & Tononi, 2014). The way we use our brains changes it, for instance, our occupation, such as London taxi drivers (Maguire et al., 2006) or attentional techniques like meditation (Muehsam et al., 2007), or pregnancy and the transition to motherhood have all been linked to changes in the structure and function of the brain. Two points should be highlighted here: first, despite the fact that brain plasticity has its limits, we now understand that the structure and activity of the brain are dynamically modified by experiences and use from early childhood into old age. Second, it may be inferred that brain plasticity is a crucial factor that shapes human culture not just in the formative years but also throughout the lifespan. The environments that are culturally mediated and in which we are raised have a crucial role in the development of our brains' functional capacities. Skills and "habits of the mind" shaped by culture take into account continuing dynamics of interaction with our local settings, niches, and the larger social ecologies we live in, in addition to neurodevelopmental processes. Consequently, our distinct brain networks become fine-tuned by daily activities and social interactions. Thoughts are formed and modified within culturally structured activities including bodily experiences. The embodiment of cultural meanings is a process carried out by our bodies and brains in the external environment, but it is not a process that our bodies or brains do independently. The ability to recognize patterns and interpret them as representations is an acquired cultural skill. The study of the meaning of human existence is hermeneutical, or a question of self-interpretation. In line with his argument, hermeneutical study is only feasible because humans, by their nature, are interpretive. Consequently, the investigation into the human existence is carried out by our own efforts to comprehend our own existence, as we interpret our existence through the course of our actions. According to Gadamer once I comprehend something, I do not just perceive it as a new concept. Rather, I experience what I have understood as something that holds truth. Consequently, hermeneutic phenomenology serves as the means that allows us to uncover, establish, and bring forth our comprehension of lived experience and existence in the world. Hermeneutic phenomenological work involves a cyclical and open approach to understand the information shared by participants in interviews, the person doing the hermeneutic phenomenological work, and ultimately, the phenomena that emerges as a result of the analysis. What emerges is a figure of hermeneutical back and forth intentional, reflective movement between what appeared, the manner of appearing and part and whole, as a path to unfold meaning. Meaning that is encountered and grasped through a practical, relational, and embodied, being-in-the world attitude.

Organization of the book

The book is organized into the following chapters that will try to answer the questions raised. Chapter 1: Solo motherhood: ART, politics, religion, and medical practice. In this chapter, the contexts are analyzed in which my grandmother belonging to a generation born at the beginning of the 20th century in Spain became a single mother in the early 1940s, and I – her granddaughter –who became a solo mother by choice with ART in the 21st century. The aim is to achieve a transgenerational view of solo motherhood in Spain, to look at which contexts it arises in, how it changes with the introduction of ART, and how the role of religion in Spanish society permeates medical practice and affects the lives of women patients. I examine two interconnected themes: (1) being a mother and being mothered are both permeated with sociocultural, political, religious, economic, and psychological significance; (2) Spain led Europe in multiple births due to ART, and ethical issues and patient rights are analyzed.

Chapter 2: Transcending blood, genes, and the biological nuclear family. The purpose of this chapter is threefold: (1) to examine the conceptualization of the links between the social and the biological in societies of the Global North, and to analyze the assumptions that implicitly underpin the literature on new forms of family, in particular, solo mothers by choice with donor-conceived children taking into account the analysis of ethnographic interviews that I have conducted during my fieldwork in Spain and in the United Kingdom; (2) to interrogate the discourses that categorize this group of women who have chosen to be mothers; and (3) to suggest a new research agenda building on the critical insights produced from addressing the first and second aims.

Chapter 3: Science, profits, and success rates. What about patient care? The purpose of this chapter is to examine the relationship between (1) the use of reproductive medicine as a business; (2) the role played by assisted reproduction clinics and their marketing strategies; and (3) the experiences of women as patients/clients. Some of the participants travelled internationally to leading reproductive destinations because of waiting lists, donor availability, success rates, cost, the anonymity of donors or embryos available to transfer, and some of them imported gametes. Reproductive treatment is not only a physiological endeavor it is also a psychological one. Despite the fact that the literature on mental health has established that psychological support is necessary in reproductive treatment, none of the women interviewed was offered this support. However, both public and private healthcare and all the industries involved in ART profit from the vast amount of money that the fertility business produces in both countries, ignoring the needs of patients.

Chapter 4: Reproductive agency and ART: the role of hospitals, legal frameworks, and the media. In this chapter, I examine the process that begins when women decide to undergo treatment with ART in private clinics (having been denied access to ART in public hospitals), how they handle the treatment, how they imagine their gestation and childbirth, their descriptions of giving birth in public hospitals, and the treatment that the obstetric teams give them. The sociocultural construction of mothers' age and of choosing a family with the help of ART, condition and bias the perception of this population in the legislative, medical, social, and media discourses.

Chapter 5: The intersection of reproductive, work–life balance, and early-education and care policies. This chapter focuses on how women's access to ART in the National Health Service was affected because they were aged 35 years or older, forcing them to go to private clinics for their treatment. Having given birth to their children, the participants face a second obstacle: the lack of policies that support work–life balance. A third obstacle also arises, in the form of a lack of childcare and early-education provision, particularly in the United Kingdom. The last two obstacles affect the whole population, but they are intensified in the case of solo-mother families where the mother is responsible for simultaneously being the care-giver and the sole economic provider. Solo motherhood by choice highlights the impact of the absence of these policies, and the inequalities that result from current contemporary conceptualizations of family, woman, and early-childhood care and education. The aim is to provide an analysis capable of capturing and confronting how inequalities affect women mothers-workers and their children.

Chapter 6: Children's education. Does feminism matter? The aim of this chapter is to analyze and compare the experiences of self-labelled feminist and non-feminist women who have consciously chosen to be solo mothers with the help of ART. The principal argument of this chapter is based on four central themes developed from the data: (1) the women participating in this study have opted to be solo mothers by choice because they have not found a suitable partner; (2) being solo mothers by choice has, for all of them, entailed a transgressive and empowering decision with regard to the traditional nuclear family; (3) the feminist participants anchor their decision to be a solo-mother family by choice in their feminism, which is also reflected in the critical pedagogy that they practice in their children's education and in the choice of secular schooling; and (4) for the non-feminist participants, the empowering and emancipatory aspect of being a solo mother by choice, their educational level, professional success, and economic independence do not have an impact on their patriarchal beliefs, and prefer Catholic or Anglican schools for their children.

Chapter 7: Conclusions. This book provides a comprehensive analysis of the process involved in becoming a solo mother through ART, starting from the age of around 35 and onwards in Spain and the United Kingdom. That is, the decision-making process, interactions with healthcare professionals and fertility clinics, the fertility industry, public policies regarding access to reproductive technology, managing the balance between work and personal life, childcare, early childhood education, and children's schooling. The book's objectives revolved around three main themes. First, I analyzed the phenomenon of becoming a solo mother focusing on the use of ART. The second theme explored the role of motherhood and examined how power is exerted through particular social institutions and cultural ideas. In the third theme I examined solo motherhood by choice and its relationship with reproductive technology as a catalyst for social change.

References

ESHRE (2017). Cross border reproductive care. www.eshre.eu/Press-Room/Resources

FecunMed (2019). España se sitúa en el tercer puesto a nivel mundial en fecundación in vitro [Spain ranks third globally in terms of in vitro fertilisation]. www.fecunmed.com/blog/espana-se-situa-en-el-tercer-puesto-a-nivel-mundial-en-fecundacion-in-vitro/

Haraway, D. J. (1991). *Simians, cyborgs, and women: The reinvention of nature*. London: Free Association Books.

Kramer, S. (2019). U.S. has world's highest rate of children living in single-parent households. www.pewresearch.org/short-reads/2019/12/12/u-s-children-more-likely-than-children-in-other-countries-to-live-with-just-one-parent/

1 Solo motherhood

ART, politics, religion, and medical practice

The case of Spain

In the case of Spain, most single-parent families are headed by women (79.1%) (Eurostat, 2015). In recent decades, there has been a dramatic increase in the number of single-parent families; the proportion of unmarried women giving birth over the age of 30 years increased from 19.9% to 46.2% (INE, 2014). And the number of single mothers by choice has increased fourfold in the last seven years (Maestro, 2015). To explore these questions, it is worth considering how motherhood is conceptualized in contemporary Spanish society. Two related issues dominate popular discourse about motherhood: (1) the difficulties of balancing work and mother-hood or rather, the incorporation of paid employment as part of what it means to be a modern Spanish mother; and (2) the fact that mothers are having their first children later in life. Spain, along with a number of southern European countries (Greece and Italy), has one of the highest gender employment gaps in the European Union. Spain is a society that can be categorized as a "traditional care model" of childcare services in which the family itself represents the main source of support (SIRC, 2012, p. 4). These types of societies are characterized by limited early childcare services and low maternal participation in the labor market. Family comes at the cost of a competitive edge in the labor market. In fact, for Spanish mothers not spending time with their families is perceived as a mark of "disadvantage", above and beyond the potential economic disadvantages of not working. Historically, the Francoist and Catholic State (1936–1975) created a patriarchal legislation, based on the authority of the husband and the father. The Francoist laws equated the family to legally constituted matrimony according to Canon Law; children produced outside of marriage were considered illegitimate. The family was the natural destination for women and the state recognized the husband as the only valid interlocutor between family and society. The ideological essence of the Franco regime was that Spain represented the spiritual haven of the West, making women the guardians of the home and tradition. In the current democracy, the 2006 law for assisted reproduction signified a change in the traditional human procreative process and in the conception of the family, since it meant giving prominence to the will of the person to freely make their life choices. However, according to data from 2010, Spain led Europe in multiple births due to assisted reproduction,

DOI: 10.4324/9781003269755-2

with the associated risks these types of births imply. Faced with the avalanche of multiple pregnancies, embryonic reduction techniques have been developed, thus creating ethical conflicts and situations lacking clarification in law. From an auto-ethnographic perspective, the subject of study is approached by analyzing the context whose understanding emerges from an implied dialogue in terms of examining the interrelations between researcher and context in order to inform and illustrate social change.

Contexts in which the decision to be a solo mother was made

In 2010, I was single and alone, making the decision that I wanted to have a child, weighing by myself the pros and cons of such a decision, when my mother asked: "Why do you want to have a child? You're just fine as you are, you've got your job, you can do what you want … to think how much work having a child is!" I thought about proclaiming that the fact that my grandmother, her mother, had been a single mother was a worthy achievement, an act of bravery in the 1940s, the decade my mother was born, a time beset by Francoism, after the civil war, and with economic hardship – although she always said that they had never lacked for food. Against all odds, my grandmother had been a single mother, although not by choice: apparently, for eight years she had been going out with a man from a higher social class than hers and the marriage could not take place, even though a child, my mother, was born to the couple. Because of this, naïve as I was, I believed that my mother would think highly of my being a solo mother through my own choice, and that she, as the daughter of a single mother, would be able to empathize with me. Yet my mother could not support my decision because she did not agree with it. Neither did she agree with my view of the empowerment of being a solo mother by choice, because she had lived through the shame of her mother being unmarried, which was perhaps a taint on the family that had to conceal it. I had come to discover that my mother was the daughter of a single mother because when I was 14 I read my mother's national identity document, and saw that the space where the name of my mother's father (my grandfather) should appear was blank, crossed out by a dashed line. So I asked my father, who was always willing to answer my questions, what this meant. He replied that my mother had no father and he told me the details, which my mother had told him before their marriage so that he would know, in case it proved a problem for him to get married to a woman who had no legal father, that is, who was an illegitimate child. My father warned me not to say anything about our conversation to my mother or to my grandmother, as they did not like to speak of it.

So that was how I found out, whispering with my father, a fact that had been hidden away in the biographies of my mother and grandmother. In all the years that my grandmother lived with us, we never talked of anything that might touch on my mother's paternity or on my grandmother's unhappy love story. Never. It was a void veiled with invisibility that weighed upon my mother, and I imagine on my grandmother too, although I never knew about it. The silence was telling. Neither did I ever hear a word against the man who had made my grandmother pregnant nor a suggestion that he should have taken responsibility for the pregnancy and, ultimately, for the creation of a new life, that of my mother. These events took place under the Franco dictatorship, whose ideology will be explained in the next section.

Women under Francoism

Sexist attitudes seeped out from the Franco era into my primary and secondary education: the woman must be protected, she must maintain her decency, she must not be a loose woman, she must make herself respected, "giving her body" is the ultimate: it is offered after getting married, when the man has respected you, has waited, has shown he loves you ... then he attains the trophy of your virginity. The Francoist laws equated the family to legally constituted matrimony according to Canon Law such that legal protection was only given to those families that were legally recognized. Thus, any other form of family relationship that was not legitimate was not only denied any protection but also, in many cases, was penalized, as in the suppositions of adultery. Moreover, the consequences of this regime fell directly on the children, who, depending on whether they had been born inside or outside of wedlock, enjoyed more or fewer rights. The system of filiation was utterly discriminatory, for civil law did not recognize illegitimate children and did not allow investigation into paternity. In the legitimate family, the Spanish state recognized the father as the only valid interlocutor between family and society. Both wife and underage children were subject to the father's authority, and the age of majority was increased to 25 years, obliging young women to stay in the paternal home until they got married or entered a convent (Iglesias de Usel, 1991).

The Franco regime particularly controlled and repressed the sexual behavior of women. The Catholic religion permeated all law, including criminal law, and therefore law was used to moralize, being oriented towards repression and not towards the protection of citizens' rights, particularly women. The Francoist criminal laws equated women with the legally unfit, and only gave protection to those women who were considered "honorable", for if they were not perceived in this way, they were treated as mere objects, at the male's disposal, who could even rape his wife without fear of criminal sanction. Everything in this matter revolved around honor, reputation, and virtue; but what was being protected was the honor of the husband and the father, not that of the woman (Cámara Villar, 1984; Instituto de la Mujer, 1985). Moreover, the penal code stated that, in the case of rape, if the forgiveness of the victim was obtained then the criminal act was expunged, thus exempting the rapist from all punishment, who could in this way avoid prison. He could also avoid prison if he married the victim. Only in 1963 did the Decree of 21st March remove what was known as "blood vengeance" from the penal code: this was the right of a father to kill his daughter or a husband his wife, along with the man who was maintaining sexual relations with her, when they were surprised committing adultery. The use of contraceptives was also explicitly punishable by law (Loree Enders, 1998). Similarly, the penal code punished abortion, both the person who carried it out and the woman who consented to have it done, except if the abortion were brought about to cover up dishonor, in which case the sentence was lesser. In the event of infanticide perpetrated by the mother or by the maternal grandparents of a newly born, conceived illegitimately and so with the purpose of hiding the dishonor, the sentence was reduced since the motive of the crime was to cover up dishonor. Nevertheless, this type of punishment could only be seen when the woman was single, widowed, or married, as long as she was respectable, because if not then the offence was classified as infanticide (Moraga García, 2008).

Under Francoism, the family model as the natural primary unit and the foundation of all society was consolidated, giving the woman the role of wife and mother. Accordingly, among her functions was to educate her children in the Catholic faith and in the Falangist doctrine, and to be the source of comfort and rest for the husband. Starting from this premise, the Francoist and Catholic state drew up a patriarchal legislation, based on the authority of the husband and father that was discriminatory for women. Thus, Spain became an example of absolute patriarchy, in which women were relegated to a position of subordination that shut them away in the domestic sphere. This legal situation, clearly inegalitarian for the woman, lasted the 40 years of the dictatorship, with barely any modification (Durán & Gallego, 1986; Nash, 1991).

The reason behind maintaining this discrimination against women is linked with the ideological essence of the regime, which was convinced that Spain was the "spiritual haven of the West" and therefore must uphold the sacred function that this regime reserved for women, of the guardians of the home and of traditional values (Bravo-Moreno, 2006, p. 71). In this ideological setting, my grandmother offered the trophy of her virginity without securing matrimony and, to add insult to injury, gave birth to an illegitimate child. This context, weighing as it does upon my mother, contaminated our conversations in which I made clear my wish to get pregnant through assisted reproduction technology (ART) in the 21st century, 70 years after my grandmother's pregnancy and the birth of my mother, in a very different historical, political, and sociocultural context. In the next section, the changes that are produced with regard to the political regime, the transformation in the concept of family, and the legal framework that allows assisted reproduction are examined.

Women and democracy

Throughout the last almost 50 years, not only have the ways of forming a family diversified, but also the internal organization of families, particularly the way in which economic responsibilities are distributed, is undergoing a profound change. The family model called "traditional", based on the division of roles and tasks between husband and wife, paid work assigned to the man and the unpaid work to the woman, is in decline. According to the 2016 census (INE, 2017), couples with both members working have come to be the majority compared with couples in which only the man works (43.6% and 27.8%, respectively). However, this transformation of the economic basis of households has not translated into a more equal joint familial responsibility in carrying out housework and childcare (González &

Jurado, 2009, p. 53). In terms of the reproductive patterns of families, Spanish women are among those who have the least children in the world, one of the lowest in the European Union (1.19 live births per woman) (Eurostat, 2021), and also among those that start to have them at an older age (the average age of having a first child is 31.6 years for women and 33.5 years for men). Although the majority of non-marital births occur to cohabiting couples and, therefore, in a familial context analogous to that of a married couple, there is also a significant percentage of births to mothers who do not cohabit with a partner in the home and who therefore constitute one-parent family units. In 2012, "single"-mother births represented 42% of all non-marital births and 16% of the total of births. Moreover, the relative proportion of these births in the whole birth rate has significantly increased in recent years: they have gone from representing 10% of total births in 2007 to 16% in 2012. In this group of mothers who do not cohabit with a partner, two subgroups probably converge: one of mothers with unplanned pregnancies and the other of solo mothers by choice. Given the increase in the prevalence of contraception in the single population (Castro Martín, 2005), one can assume that a large proportion of solo-mother pregnancies are intentional. The fact that 56% of the births to mothers without a cohabiting partner are to women above the age of 30 years suggests that a significant proportion of these births are the result of careful decision. Secularization, the rise in the divorce rate and in one-parent families, which have increased the social visibility of solo mothers, have probably contributed to increasing the acceptance of solo motherhood as an option. In the following section, I explore my personal experience in the process of becoming a mother using ART.

Assisted reproduction technology: my own journey

Once I had taken the decision that I wished to be a mother regardless of whether I had the support or not of my own mother, I went ahead. In the private assisted reproduction clinic, they told me that my age would not be a problem. The law on assisted reproduction passed in 2006 provided for the possibility of being a mother until the age of 50 if done privately, though only until 35 years old if done through public healthcare.

ART has brought about a change in the traditional human procreative process and in the conception of the family (Franklin and McKinnon, 2002; Strathern, 1992). It has meant giving special prominence to the will of a person. The connection between procreation and the free development of personality, enshrined in Article 10.1 of the Spanish Constitution, is obvious, when understanding this constitutional principle as the autonomy of a person to freely and responsibly select the life choices that are most in line with their preferences (Berrocal Lanzarot, 2007). In this law, the decision as to how many oocytes can be fertilized is left to the judgment of the doctor. However, in the case of in vitro fertilization (IVF) and similar techniques, the transfer of a maximum of three pre-embryos only in each woman in each reproductive cycle is authorized, in order to avoid multiple pregnancies (BOE, 2006, art. 3, section 2). In the cases of assisted fertilization with the contribution of a donor or donors, the child born as a result holds legal filiation from the biological mother and her partner (if one exists), when "they have given their previous and express formal consent" to this type of fertilization, and neither the woman who gives birth (nor her partner) may contest the legally determined filiation. Therefore, the child is awarded the status of legitimate child when the genetic material employed is not from either of the spouses (BOE, 2006, art. 8, section 1).

My interest in the topic of ART originated when I lived in London and at the age of 38 years I attended a conference sponsored by a private assisted reproduction clinic in which egg vitrification was discussed. At the age of 39 years I moved to Spain and decided to freeze my eggs. I began to investigate which clinics had more prestige and more experience in assisted reproduction, and the IVI Clinic was a solid option, so I traveled to their headquarters in Valencia, in 2004. They assigned me a young gynecologist who informed me that I could freeze my eggs and have access to them when I decided to get pregnant. I understood by doing this that I would significantly enhance my prospects of conceiving in the future. The gynecologist did not explain that vitrifying my eggs before the age of 35 would have increased the success rate by 40% compared with freezing them later. Moreover, the best time to preserve fertility is before the age of 35, after that age the quality of the eggs is no longer as good, which decreases the chances of a future pregnancy. In the case of women between 36 and 40 years of age, fertility decreases dramatically and there is a high risk of chromosomal alterations in the eggs. This information, currently shown on the clinic's website, was not disclosed to me by the gynecologist I consulted nearly two decades ago when I started my journey to conceive.

After my first visit to the clinic I underwent a gynecological examination and received a prescription for ovarian stimulation. Treatment began with the menstrual cycle, lasting between 10 and 12 days. It consisted of the administration of hormone injections that stimulated the development of multiple eggs within each ovary. When the number and size of the eggs were adequate, a dose of the hormone hCG, which induced ovulation, was administered and the puncture was scheduled in the clinic 36 hours later. Thus, I self-administered daily injections of prescribed hormones on my belly. The overall expenses, including prescribed vitamin complexes and clinical tests, amounted to nearly €2,000. Every day at the same time in the afternoon I injected myself with hormones, wherever I was. If I were strolling down the street, I would enter a cafeteria's bathroom to inject myself with the medication. The aspiration of the eggs was performed in the operating room and under total anesthesia. In the puncture procedure, which lasted around 20 minutes, the ovaries were accessed through the vagina, from where the eggs were aspirated and collected in tubes, so they were taken to the IVF laboratory, where they were vitrified. After the procedure, I was in the hospital for a while until I was discharged. They informed me that the ovarian stimulation had resulted in eight oocytes that were treated with protective means for freezing, so that they would not suffer any damage in the cooling process. Once the process was finished, they were placed on small supports that were immersed in liquid nitrogen, at a temperature of –196°C.

When I was 45 years old I returned to the same clinic to have my eggs and semen from my then partner used. Thus, the two eggs that had the highest quality were chosen to be inseminated and IVF was performed under general anesthesia. I had two embryos transferred at Christmas 2010, but a few weeks later after a check-up they told me I was not pregnant. I had lost the possibility of becoming a mother with my own eggs since I was informed that the rest of the oocytes were not of good quality. I was overwhelmed with deep sadness. The gynecologist who had treated me was attending an international conference and sent me an email stating that the risk of not conceiving had materialized. I lost the possibility of conceiving with my own eggs and the gynecologist did not provide me with any guidance regarding the psychological and emotional impact of losing my two embryos. His role as a gynecologist specialized in ART had ended. As if it were a sealed compartment: the reproductive treatment had not resulted in success, end of story. It felt as if my reproductive system and my mind were separated and did not inhabit the same body. I found his interaction mediated by an e-mail dehumanizing. I lost the possibility of conceiving with my eggs and what did I do with the emotions that shook me?

The relationship with my partner ended, but I continued with my desire to be a mother. Added to the desolation of not being able to be a mother with my eggs was the sadness that my relationship had ended. My family doctor told me that access to reproductive treatment at the NHS was only for women up to the age of 35 years. He could perform some tests on me, nothing else. I began to investigate local clinics in the small town where I lived, in one of them they told me that they offered the treatment only to heterosexual couples with fertility problems. Another private clinic, where research was also carried out, offered me confidence, and also the possibility of having a session with a psychologist specialized in assisted reproduction. The psychologist told me that I was experiencing two bereavements: the genetic grief and also the sadness for the breakup of my relationship. She gave a name to what I felt and that I did not know existed: genetic grief.

I was clear that I only wanted to have one baby, since I was alone in that city, I had no family network or friends who could help me. And I only wanted to undergo a cycle of assisted reproduction that, according to the clinic, involved two attempts; if the second attempt did not result in a live baby, I would have to pay for another cycle. In the following section, I examine the processes of assisted reproduction clinics, through which solo mothers by choice necessarily pass, and the ethical challenges that both professional health workers and women must face.

ART and multiple births

When it came to my decision to have a child, I knew that ART was not so sophisticated as to be able to respect my wish of having just one baby and not a multiple pregnancy. This has been the case for too many families that wished to have just one child through assisted reproduction, for whom the treatment resulted in several gestational sacs, in other words, in the possible result of having two or more babies. In my case, I was clear that I could only have one: I was alone, I had no family network that might help me, and economically I could comfortably maintain one child but would have extreme difficulties with more than one. Bearing this in mind, I informed the doctor and director of the assisted reproduction clinic. She told me that this would not be a problem. The technique was indeed not so precise as to be able to choose beforehand the number of children desired. However, there was a technique that refined the treatment, which was called "embryonic reduction". Once I began the treatment, it was successful straight away, so much so that two gestational sacs were found in my uterus. Delighted by the success but worried by the double success, while remembering my conversation with the clinic's director, I went to her for a solution. As she was not in the clinic, a gynecologist and obstetrician attended to me. He was university professor, researcher, and national award winner for contraception. When I requested a solution, this doctor reacted with surprise. He said that I must have known what to expect when I underwent the assisted reproductive treatment that there was the chance that more than one embryo would be successfully implanted and that, therefore, he could not offer me anything as a result. When I insisted that the director of the clinic had assured me that if more than one embryo was successful, an embryonic reduction could be done, the doctor blurted out that he was a Catholic and because of his religious beliefs he could not give me that option. The nurse was witness to my surprise and discomfort. There I was, facing a man who decided when to play at being God[1] – making the fertilization of embryos possible – and when to play the Catholic, censuring the possibility of correcting an error derived from assisted reproductive treatment. When a medical doctor subjects the life of another human being to moral judgment, he disregards the individual who is, de facto, practicing her or his own specific ethical code. The doctor, from his supposed universal reason, which is really his own personal reason shored up in powerful institutional and religious devices, wrests individuals' own personal leadership as ethical agents from them, in a sort of enlightened despotism. Dov Fox, professor of law at San Diego University, asserts that:

> The best way for courts to think about this new right is in terms of whether professional wrongdoing (1) imposes unwanted procreation, (2) deprives wanted procreation, or (3) confounds plans either to have or to avoid having offspring, not just of any type, but with traits that parents project would make their experience of raising a child more worthwhile or less gratifying … . Where the law weighs in on conflicts about selective procreation, it should give voice to the conflicting sentiments that pervade it. But these concerns don't justify categorically treating professional misconduct in procreation as a vicissitude of life no different from a spontaneous miscarriage or roll of the genetic dice. These transgressions are wrongs in need of a right.
>
> (2016)

Needless to say, I left the clinic extremely worried, not knowing what to do. I had so much wanted to be a mother, to the extent of going to a clinic of assisted reproduction and receiving hormone treatment, sedation, fertilization, and going through all the stages that may result in an embryo, but which actually produced two. The contradiction passed through my mind that having got pregnant through ART, I now saw myself in the obligation of interrupting the pregnancy because I could not have more than one baby. With this worry, and anger at the contradiction of two doctors belonging to the same clinic, one the director and the other her employee, I immediately called the clinic to arrange an appointment with her, the doctor and clinic director who had assured me that they could remedy the error in the ART. In the appointment, I stated what the doctor had argued. The director had already heard a version from the nurse of the dialectical clash between the doctor and myself. She told me that there was no problem, but that I would have to go to another city, to a clinic where they carried out embryonic reductions. She had already called the clinic and they were expecting me. In her clinic, they did not perform that type of procedure … due to religious reasons.

Legality, ethical conflicts, and patient rights

The rate of multiple gestations has significantly increased in recent decades, the main reason being the use of ART. Faced with the avalanche of multiple gestations, embryonic reduction techniques have been developed aimed at improving perinatal survival and reducing the risks to the mother, thus creating ethical conflicts and situations not completely clarified by the existent legislation (Dickens & Cook, 2008). The technique of embryonic reduction reduces the number of gestational sacs, with the aim of increasing the possibilities that gestation reaches full term and, therefore, promoting fetal viability. The recognition of the practice of embryonic reduction within assisted reproduction was reflected in Law 2003 section 45 (BOE, 2003), replaced by Law 2006 section 14, while the law on voluntary interruption of pregnancy must also be taken into account, currently constituted by Organic Law 2010 section 2 (Guisado Fernández et al., 2015). Social, economic, and emotional motives have an influence on deciding for embryonic reduction. The Committee for the Ethical Aspects of Human Reproduction and Women's Health (FIGO, 2006) and the American College of Obstetricians and Gynecologists (2013) state that this option can be offered depending on the patient, medical factors and the social, psychological, and economic circumstances that determine the final decision. The situation under consideration must be implicitly categorized on what is deemed the justifying state of necessity (art. 20, section 5 of the Spanish Penal Code), this being the mechanism for ruling out its punishability (Abellán & Sánchez-Caro, 2009; Evans et al., 2001).

In my own case, both the procedure of assisted reproduction and that of embryonic reduction were separate financial costs, on top of the amount paid for the treatment: paying for hormones, blood analyses, and gynecological tests; a bill that I was able to meet with my salary but I was fully aware that a woman with lesser means would not be able to afford it. Thus, my wishes to be a mother were conditioned by my economic status. I was also conscious that if my finances had meant that I could not afford the treatment and the long-term raising of my child, I would not have wanted to bring a life into this world. I did not believe it would be responsible of me: I did not wish to bring a child into a life of hardship but into one of economic capability within which other possibilities could originate. In Article 4 of Law 2006 section 14, it lays down that as a preliminary to the starting treatment, the medical team must analyze the situation of each woman or each couple, seeing whether, considering their specific reproductive case, they can meet those aspects of the treatment. In order to do this, the woman's particular circumstances are considered, such as her age, clinical history, and the possible causes of sterility. Iriberri (2011) states that reducing the number of multiple pregnancies has become an objective for experts in assisted reproduction. In every conference, there are many studies of new strategies to improve the success of assisted reproductive techniques without having to resort to implanting two or three embryos, the maximum permitted by law. In Spain, there are more and more multiple births despite the decrease in the overall number of births. In 2014, the Spanish National Institute of Statistics (INE) recorded 9,612 childbirths of more than one baby, 2.2% of the total. This should be compared with the rest of European countries, where "the average fluctuates between 1 and 1.5%", explains María de la Calle, gynecologist at the Multiple Gestations Unit of the public La Paz Hospital in Madrid. In only 10 years, multiple births have increased almost 20.5%, even though the total number of births has reduced to 6.4%. And the growth from 18 years ago has increased 110%: there are now double the number of multiple births than almost two decades ago (Iriberri, 2011). Spain is the leader in multiple births, according to the European Perinatal Health Report, published in 2013 with data from 2010 (Euro-Peristat Project with SCPE and EUROCAT, 2013) and one of the causes of this, apart from maternity in advanced age, is that up to three embryos can legally be transferred in IVF, whereas in the Scandinavian countries this is limited to one.

Despite the scope of the phenomenon, the data on assisted reproduction are partial, since up until now public hospitals and private clinics were not obliged to make their statistics public. There is no register of multiple families, and neither Institute of National Statistics (INE), which does record single-parent homes, nor the Ministry of Health, which does have a census of large families, takes it into account. In order to find out how many multiple families there are, one must turn to the INE (Spanish National Institute of Statistics) tables of births. If all the children from multiple births lived in the same city along with their parents, they would fill the sixth largest city in Spain, Málaga, by number of inhabitants, with a total of 572,947 people (Census, 2015). If the implantation of two embryos improves the success rates of assisted reproductive techniques, which many women turn to over at the age of 35 when their possibilities of having children are naturally lower, there nevertheless is a determination to avoid it since, as Antonio Requena, medical director of one of the busiest private clinics in Spain, states: "The human species is made to have single births; it is documented that there is greater obstetric pathology among women pregnant with twins" (Iribarri, 2011). As López Sastre remarks, the big problem with twin births, beyond the fact that women have a more complicated pregnancy, is the increase in premature children (Aguilar, 2016). The director of the Stem Cell Bank of the Barcelona Center of Regenerative Medicine, Anna Veiga, agrees that the top current aim of assisted reproduction is "the decrease in multiple pregnancies". Veiga states that the Nordic countries are the leaders in this respect. Requena believes that this is because their social security covers many more cycles of treatment than in other countries (an average of four, as opposed to two in Spain) and, moreover, there is no waiting list. This is why they can permit the single transfer, even though the success rate is, in principle, lower (Guisado Fernández et al., 2015).

In 2024, the European Society of Human Reproduction and Embryology (ESHRE) published a guideline on the number of embryos to transfer during IVF/ICSI (in vitro fertilization and intracytoplasmic sperm injection, respectively) based on the collected evidence, recommendations were discussed until a consensus was reached within the Guideline Development Group (GDG) and the final version was approved by the GDG and the ESHRE Executive Committee. They concluded that single embryo transfer is the preferred method for safe and successful ART. Currently, this is endorsed by numerous worldwide and national professional organizations. In Europe, there was a reduction in the use of double embryo transfer and an increase in the choice transfer of a single embryo at a time. Nevertheless, the results indicate a significant disparity in the implementation of single embryo transfer, with varying levels of adherence to guidelines across different countries. ESHRE (2024) recommends the single embryo transfer for financial issues of multiple pregnancy/birth: (1) increased direct costs related to obstetric care of multiple pregnancies and pediatric care of twins and triplets; (2) increased indirect costs with multiple pregnancies due to sick leave days, over-the-counter medication, and loss of productivity because of an ill child. The GDG recommends that cost-related information should be provided and discussed with the patient(s) at the treatment planning stage. In addition, the ESHRE guideline (2024) recommends single embryo transfer due to psychological issues of multiple pregnancy/birth, that is, clinicians should consider the possible complications of multiple pregnancies with regards to mental health: postpartum, emotional distress, as well as the influence of personality characteristics, sociodemographic factors, and family functioning, on the mental health of parents and offspring regardless of the number of children born. The GDG also recommends that information on possible psychosocial complications should be provided to patients at the treatment planning stage (ESHRE, 2024, p. 4). Moreover, the ESHRE guideline argues that using a double embryo transfer should be avoided for procedures involving donor oocytes, donated embryos, or gestational carriers due to significantly higher risks of pregnancy problems, and a single embryo transfer is strongly recommended for these cases. Thus, the ESHRE guideline concludes that the following issues are crucial for decision-making regarding the number of embryos to transfer and how they should be discussed with the patient(s): (1) medical, economic, social, and psychological consequences of transferring more than one embryo; (2) patient wishes regarding family building, and (c) clinical, science-based recommendations for the specific patient case. Apart from counselling on the potential pregnancy difficulties associated with transferring more than one embryo and the consequent multiple gestations, patients considering double embryo transfer should be informed that the likelihood of ectopic pregnancy rises proportionally with the quantity of embryos transferred, up to approximately 20 times higher, independent of their stage of development or whether they have been frozen. Furthermore, a singleton pregnancy resulting from a double embryo transfer is linked to an increased risk of neonatal death and poor birth-weight in frozen embryo transfer, compared with a single pregnancy following a single embryo transfer (ESHRE, 2024).

Needless to say I was never informed of any issues the ESHRE guidelines (2024) refer to in its latest report by any of the clinics I visited, or by the specialists in ART that talked at the events sponsored by the fertility industry I attended till 2021. The women I interviewed for this study in Spain and the United Kingdom had not been informed either.

My request for embryonic reduction made to the clinic director did not prove to be so simple. I had not been informed of the religious directives of the clinic that treated me. Some pressure groups, such as American Atheists in the United States (Atheist.org, 2015), believe that there should be a law entitled the "Patient's Right to Know", which would require medical service providers to inform patients of their religious inclinations.

I came up against a Catholic doctor, in this society where the recognition of religious freedom appears to justify the refusal to perform his job, that is, the purpose for which he was paid: to produce one, single, viable fetus. In this society, the possibility that religion pervades the praxis of doctors, pharmacists, hospitals, or clinics is real. Patient rights require that, if medical treatment or information that would otherwise be available to the patient is withheld based on religious beliefs, then the healthcare provider in question must inform the patient of this in writing. As other authors (Giesen, 1993, p. 554; Gillon, 1994, p. 177) have argued before, there should be legislation regarding the patient's right to know, which would require medical professionals and pharmacists who refuse to provide a service for religious reasons to give written notice to patients, listing all the services to which the patient will not have access due to such reasons. Patients should be able to make fully informed decisions about their health. A woman who wants contraceptive pills, for example, and goes to the doctor for the prescription, or to the pharmacist to sell them to her, does not deny the right of that doctor or that pharmacist to practice their religion. Moreover, both doctors and pharmacists should avoid giving moral condemnation and refusing to prescribe or sell contraceptives.

Therefore, requiring that healthcare clinics and providers disclose their religious inclinations is the best protection for patients and users (Rubin Erdely, 2007b). In a survey published in 2007 by the *New England Journal of Medicine*, 63% of doctors said that it was acceptable to tell patients that they objected morally to certain treatments and 18% felt no obligation to refer patients to another medical center (Farr et al., 2007). Jamie Brooks, a former attorney with the National Health Law Program who continues working on projects with the advocacy group, asserts that "doctors swear an oath to serve their patients. But instead, they are allowing their religious beliefs to compromise patient care. And too often, the victims of this practice are women" (Rubin Erdely, 2007a). Compared with the number of pharmacists who refuse to dispense contraceptives or the morning-after pill, the number of doctors that do not prescribe a treatment that goes against their beliefs is less visible. Patients who are refused treatment rarely complain because the situation tends to be personally humiliating and when patients do make a fuss, the cases are resolved on the quiet.

In the case of Madrid in the first decade of the 21 century, an abortion request for reasons of the mental health of the mother could not go ahead in public healthcare without a favorable report written by a psychiatrist. According to the social workers interviewed for a study on the reproductive health of immigrant women in Madrid (Bravo-Moreno, 2005, p. 101), only the psychiatrists from 2 healthcare areas (out of a total of 11) wrote reports in the favor of abortion due to the mental health of the mother. The women who wanted an abortion in public healthcare were referred to these two psychiatrists because in the rest of the healthcare districts, the psychiatrists always gave unfavorable reports. However, the mayor of Madrid then in power restricted this option when he decreed that only the residents of Districts A and B could have access to the services of those two psychiatrists. Thus, those women who did not live in those areas had no choice but to go to the professional corresponding to their district, who would give an unfavorable report. Consequently, a strategy was created by which a social worker in a National Health System hospital referred women without financial means to private clinics at the cost of the National Health System by using other expense concepts. In other cases, this social worker noted, there were gynecologists who refused to insert the intrauterine device and referred patients to other health centers because they felt uncomfortable with issues of family planning such as abortion or the intrauterine device.

Conclusion

Through the understanding gained from personal experience and total immersion in the field, which is essential in anthropological knowledge, I have attempted to illustrate aspects of myself, the researcher, and of the world I inhabit. With this hermeneutic circle, I have also attempted to tackle two axes: my own world and the social world that I wish to comprehend. As Wall (2006, p. 1) states: "The intent of auto-ethnography is to acknowledge the inextricable link between the personal and the cultural". In such a way that the participant observation in the politically charged context that is addressed has required negotiating between three modes of participation in reality: the emotional, the analytical, and the political, the latter dimension derived from a sense of ethical responsibility that originates in feelings of injustice towards the other and that provokes the impulse to act. Transcending in this way the idea of ethnographic fieldwork perceived as intellectual, analytical, and academic and not political and pragmatic entailing a political response.

In this chapter, I have aimed to give a trans-generational perspective on the one-parent family led by women anchored in the historical, sociocultural, political, and religious conditions of lives that were lived in the Franco dictatorship and presently in democracy. Under the Franco dictatorship and National Catholicism, the ideal family was represented with the husband as the head of the family just as God was head of the church. Yet more in accordance with these ideological parameters, the differences of gender were perceived as biological, determined in part by the celestial order; progeny produced out of canonical wedlock held no rights until 1978, when the Constitution proclaimed that all children were equal before the law, regardless of the origin of their filiation. Today, although the democratic state is officially secular, part of the medical community still reproduces visions of the past and of a present tinged by religion, thus violating women's rights. This is such that reproductive health is perceived as different to looking after regular health; it is not seen as a matter to treat but as something loaded with morality, and if professional health workers perceive it as a moral matter, it becomes something to which one can say yes or no. This has meant that doctors, despite their oath to serve their patients, allow their religious beliefs to compromise the care of their patients. All too often, those affected by these practices are women. Men, in general, escape such scrutiny: It is difficult to imagine that a doctor would think he is going to hell for requesting a vasectomy. And if there are women who fear the moral judgment of their doctors, other problems can result: it is possible that there are women who do not communicate with their doctors or avoid requesting treatment. Whatever the case, it is dangerous for women. The fact that doctors refuse to offer treatment due to their moral objections and can refer patients to another center, recalls other eras, such as those of civil rights ("I won't treat blacks, Latinos, gypsies, 'irregular' immigrants", and so on), diverting patients to another health center, and all cases of discrimination. In the case of Spain, the change of political regime, the legal framework in which assisted reproduction is practiced, and the transformation of reproductive patterns do not protect women against the discrimination that they may suffer in clinics sending them on to another center due to the religious belief of the professional health workers.

Note

1 The Apostolic Exhortation Amoris Laetitia (The Joy of Love), on love in the family, presented on 8 April 2016, brings together the results of the 2014 and 2015 synods. In the second chapter of this document, entitled "The Experiences and Challenges of Families", the Pope refers to "various forms of an ideology of gender that 'denies the difference and reciprocity in nature of a man and a woman'". The Pope calls into question assisted reproductive technologies that have "introduced the ability to manipulate the reproductive act (…). In this way, human life and parenthood have become modular and separable realities, subject mainly to the wishes of individuals or couples. (…) Let us not fall into the sin of trying to replace the Creator. We are creatures, and not omnipotent. Creation is prior to us and must be received as a gift. At the same time, we are called to protect our humanity, and this means, in the first place, accepting it and respecting it as it was created". On the vocation of the family, the Pope states that "the absence of a father gravely affects family life and the upbringing of children and their integration into society. This absence, which may be physical, emotional, psychological and spiritual, deprives children of a suitable father figure". (Retrieved from www.religionconfidencial.com/vaticano/Papa-ideolo gia-inquietante-imponerse-pensamiento_0_2688331169.html).

References

Abellán, F., & Sánchez-Caro, J. (2009). *Bioética y ley en reproducción humana asistida: Manual de casos clínicos*. Granada: Comares.

Aguilar, A. M. (2016). Los partos múltiples se duplican en España en casi dos décadas. *20 minutos*. Retrieved from www.20minutos.es/noticia/2797260/0/aumentan-nacimientos-mul tiples-espana-gemelos/

American College of Obstetricians and Gynecologists. (2013). Committee opinion no. 553: Multifetal pregnancy reduction. *Obstetrics & Gynecology, 121*, 405–410. doi: 10.1016/j.ijgo.2005.12.019

Atheist.org. (2015). Atheists demand 'right to know act' for patients in America's religious health care system. Retrieved from http://news.atheists.org/2015/09/29/atheists-dem and-right-to- know-act-for-patients-in-americas-religious-health-care-system/

Berrocal Lanzarot, A. I. (2007). Análisis de la nueva Ley 14/2006, de 26 de mayo sobre técnicas de reproducción humana asistida. Una primera aproximación a su contenido. *Revista de la Escuela de Medicina Legal*. Retrieved from http://pendientedemigracion. ucm.es/info/medlegal/ 5%20Escuelas/escumedlegal/revista/articulos_pdf/4_4_2007.pdf

BOE. (2003). Retrieved from www.boe.es/boe/dias/2003/11/22/pdfs/A41458-41463.pdf

BOE. (2006). Retrieved from www.boe.es/buscar/act.php?idDBOE-A-2006-9292

Bravo-Moreno, A. (2005). El aborto en la población inmigrante: Contextualización. In M. L. Esteban Galarza & J. Pallarés Gómez (Coord.), *La salud en una sociedad multicultural: Desigualdad, mercantilización y medicalización* (pp. 99–113). X Congreso de Antropología. Sevilla: Fundación El Monte.

Bravo-Moreno, A. (2006). *Migration, gender and national identity*. Bern: Peter Lang.

Cámara Villar, G. (1984). *Nacional-catolicismo y escuela. La socialización política del Franquismo (1931–1951)*. Jaén: Hespería.

Castro Martín, T. (2005). Contraceptive use patterns among Spanish single youth. *European Journal of Contraception and Reproductive Health Care, 10*(4), 219–228.

Census. (2015). Retrieved from www.ine.es/

Dickens, B., & Cook, R. J. (2008). Multiple pregnancy: Legal and ethical issues. *International Journal of Gynecology and Obstetrics, 103*, 270–274.

Durán, M. A., & Gallego, T. (1986). The women's movement in Spain and the new Spanish democracy. In D. Dahlerup (Ed.), *The new women's movement. Feminism and political power in Europe and the USA* (pp. 48–81). London: Sage.

ESHRE (European Society of Human Reproduction and Embryology). (2024). Guideline group on the number of embryos to transfer during IVF/ICSI. Alessandra Alteri, Gemma Arroyo, Giuliana Baccino et al. Human Reproduction. Retrieved from https://doi.org/ 10.1093/humrep/deae010

Euro-Peristat Project with SCPE and EUROCAT. (2013). European perinatal health report. The health and care of pregnant women and babies in Europe in 2010. Retrieved from www.europeristat.com/images/European%20Perinatal%20Health%20Report_2010.pdf

Eurostat. (2015). People in the EU: Statistics on household and family structures. Retrieved from http://ec.europa.eu/eurostat/statistics-explained/index.php/People_ in_the_EU_%E2%80%93_ statistics_on_household_and_family_structures

Eurostat. (2021). Fertility statistics. https://ec.europa.eu/eurostat/statistics-explained/index. php?title=Fertility_statistics#live_births_per_woman_in_the_EU_in_2021

Evans, M. I., Berkowitz, R., Wapner, R., Carpenter, R., Goldberg, J., & Ayoub, M. A., et al. (2001). Multifetal pregnancy reduction (MFPR): Improved outcomes with increased experience. *American Journal of Obstetrics & Gynecology, 184*, 97–103.

Farr, A. C., Ryan, E. L., Marshall, H., Chin, M. P. H., & Lantos, J. D. (2007). Religion, con-science, and controversial clinical practices. *New England Journal of Medicine, 356*, 593–600.
FIGO. (2006). Committee for the ethical aspects of human reproduction and women's health. Ethical recommendations on multiple pregnancy and multifetal reduction. *International Journal of Gynecology & Obstetrics, 92*(3), 331–332.
Fox, D. (2016, March 4). From chance to choice to court. [Blog post]. Retrieved from huffington post.com/dov-fox/from-chance-to-choice-to_b_9605450.html
Franklin, S., & McKinnon, S. (Eds.) (2002). *Relative values. Reconfiguring kinship studies.* Durham: Duke University Press.
Giesen, D. (1993). The patient's right to know: A comparative law perspective. *Medical Law, 12*(6–8), 553–565.
Gillon, R. (1994). Medical ethics: Four principles plus attention to scope. *British Medical Journal, 309*, 175–184.
González, M. J., & Jurado, T. (2009). Cuándo se implican los hombres en las tareas domésticas? Un análisis de la Encuesta de Empleo del Tiempo. *Panorama Social, 10*, 65–81.
Guisado Fernández, J., García Lozano, J. C., & Carrillo Vadillo, R. (2015). Aspectos éticos y legales de la gestación múltiple. Retrieved from www.hvn.es/servicios_asistencia les/ ginecologia_y_obstetricia/ficheros/actividad_docente_e_investigadora/curso_de_ actualizacion_en_obstetricia_y_ginecologia/curso_2016/obstetricia/5_aspectos_eticos_ legales_gestacion_ multiple.pdf
Iglesias de Usel, J. (1991). Family, ideology and political transition in Spain. *International Journal of Law and the Family, 5*, 277–295.
INE. (2014). Población. Retrieved from www.ine.es/prodyser/espa_cifras/2014/#2
INE. (2017). Mercado laboral. Retrieved from www.ine.es/ss/Satellite?LDes_ES&cD INEPublicacion_C&cidD1259924856416&pD1254735110672&pagenameDProductosY Servicios%2FPYSLayout&param1DPYS
Instituto de la Mujer. (1985). *El trabajo de las mujeres a través de la historia.* Madrid: Ministerio de Cultura.
Iribarri, A. (2011, September 27). La ciencia investiga cómo frenar los embarazos múltiples. *Público*. Retrieved from www.publico.es/ciencias/ciencia-investiga-frenar-embarazos-multiples.html
Loree Enders, V. (Ed.) (1998). *Constructing Spanish womanhood: Female identity in modern Spain.* New York: State University of New York Press.
Maestro, R. (2015). Aumento del número de madres solas por elección. Retrieved from http://masola.org/reproduccion-asistida-2/la-reproduccion-asist ida-en-el-punto-de-mira-de- europa/
Moraga García, M. A. (2008). Notas sobre la situación jurídica de la mujer en el Franquismo. *Feminismo/s, 12*, 229–252.
Nash, M. (1991). Pronatalism and motherhood in Franco´s Spain. In G. Bock & P. Thane (Eds.), *Maternity and gender policies: Women and rise of the European welfare states 1880s–1950s* (pp. 175–197). London: Routledge.
Rubin Erdely, S. (2007a, May 21). Could your doctor deny you health care? *Self.* Retrieved from www.self.com/story/denial-of-health-care

Rubin Erdely, S. (2007b, June 22). Doctors' beliefs can hinder patient care. *Self*. Retrieved from www.nbcnews.com/id/19190916/ns/health-womens_health/t/doctors-beliefs-can-hin der-patient-care/

SIRC (Social Issues Research Centre). (2012). The changing face of motherhood in Western Europe: Spain. Retrieved from www.sirc.org.

Strathern, M. (1992). *Reproducing the future: Essays on anthropology, kinship and the new reproductive technologies*. Manchester: Manchester University Press.

2 Transcending blood, genes, and the biological nuclear family

Does genetics make a family?

The genetic–biologistic model that associates sexuality with reproduction, reproduction with heterosexual relations, heterosexual relations with marriage, marriage with the family, and the family with the middle-class nuclear model is dependent on a chain of significations that have been rendered outdated by developments in reproductive processes (Kroløkke et al., 2015; Stone, 2013; Strathern, 1992). The symbol par excellence of this cultural kinship system is consanguinity: blood together with other biogenetic substances such as the semen and the egg that represent genealogical "legitimacy" and biological traceability as the basic component of individual identity for societies in the Global North, wealthy industrialized countries (Odeh, 2010). Sharing and passing on one's blood and genetic information as a result of the sexual act is the natural element that legitimizes the establishment of social, filial, conjugal, and fraternal relations that extend upward and downward to make the genealogical tree, the basic underlying layer of these societies' idea of kinship. This conceptualization of the links between the social and the biological, between nature and culture, is particular to the Global North (Schneider, 1980). This was the dominant trend in kinship studies until the 1960s, in which kinship was defined as the sociocultural interpretation that a group constructs out of the biological facts of reproduction. Kinship, as defined in anthropology and associated with the facts of reproduction, biology and genealogy, cannot be made universal because it is always particular to a culture in a particular context. Schneider (1984) suggested that most anthropologists had in one way or another defined kinship in relation to human biological reproduction. They did so because of an implicit and mistaken assumption, namely, that their own Western cultural notion that "blood is thicker than water" is a human universal. Schneider suggested that this idea of kinship might only exist in Euro-American society. What the biological facts of reproduction represent for American, British, or Spanish kinship can for other societies be represented by other types of practices: common, shared acts such as residing together, the eating of food, the raising of children, the land, heritage, or rituals, among other aspects (Stone, 2001). In some New Guinea groups, people became members of descent groups through common residence, reinforced by food sharing (Strathern, 1992).

DOI: 10.4324/9781003269755-3

The analysis of kinship became transformed through the incorporation of the ideas of social processes as opposed to structures; of the individual as an active agent with capacity for initiative as opposed to the conception of the individual as a simple, passive subject in structures; and of social action as deliberate action and human agency. And thus the perspective that, until that time, had prioritized kinship as a principle of social organization and integration was abandoned (Lamphere, 2001; Stone, 2001). Numerous theorists and researchers have also pointed out that power is embedded in kinship as well as in other domains such as politics, religion, ethnicity, and nation (Chodorow, 1978; Glenn et al., 1994; Okin, 1989; Phoenix et al., 1991; Rich, 1995; Yanagisako & Delaney, 1995). The new possibilities of reproduction, in vitro fertilization, gamete donation, and surrogacy, have raised new possibilities for thinking about kinship. Women themselves have confronted situations where the "biological facts" can no longer be considered "natural". For example, surrogate mothers downplay their genetic contribution and view the adoptive mother as someone who has conceived the child "in her heart" not through her body (Ragoné, 1994). These issues give rise to wider questions about how to tackle the interaction between nature and culture and how anthropology and other disciplines, such as psychology and family studies, can reproduce or question these concepts (Strathern, 1992). As cultural facts, such ideas inform our representations, descriptions, and analyses of kinship. At the same time, we envision possibilities through ideas that already exist and are part of the cultural repertoire. The premise of social anthropology is that what is taken for granted as being facts of nature are themselves sociocultural constructions (Strathern, 1992). The "natural" facts of procreation are enshrined in the law. Currently, legal parents need not be the biological or genetic father and/or mother of the baby but can be the donor of genetic material. Being a donor or providing a womb, or being the person who takes care of and educates the child, are separate things and none is sufficient by itself to produce a social, emotional, or psychological bond. A decision must be made about what type of relation is to be practiced as a consequence of the biological connection (O'Reilly, 2007; Strathern, 1992). Professor Daniels (2006), who has worked in the field of assisted human reproduction for the past 30 years and, who adopted twins with his wife, says that we have to reflect on how assisted reproduction and its impact makes us think about the meaning of "family":

> We are still stuck in a very genetic connotation that family is only a family if there's a biological link between the parents and the child and that represents something of a challenge for people like ourselves who just don't fit into that norm.
>
> (p. 266)

Another relevant issue concerning genetics is the nature versus nurture debate. "How much of children's make-up is from genes and how much from the environment they grow up in?" (Daniels, 2006, p. 63). Most mothers and fathers whose children have been conceived through the donation of genetic material agree that it is the relationship that they build with their children that is the most important.

It is not necessary to share genetic material to form an intense emotional, psychological, and emotional relationship with a child and be a good mother or father. Janet Carsten is one of the anthropologists who have most developed the concept of "relatedness" as an alternative to the term "kinship", seeking to avoid Western ideas on kinship centered on the facts of procreation and the division between the biological and the social. Her proposal is to study the emic conceptions and perceptions of the modes of establishing relations and of being related, thus enabling transcultural comparison (Carsten, 2000). Her contribution to kinship studies as a process that is constructed through daily practices has proved to be a highly useful tool when it comes to studying the current modes of becoming related in Euro-American societies, in which blood appears to have ceased to be "thicker than water", or at least seems not always to be, nor in the same way, for all social actors. The increase in divorce and successive marriages or unions with children of one or both partners, homosexual couples with children, solo parenthood, international adoption and assisted reproductive techniques, or the transnationalization of families has generated new modalities of relatedness that are stripping biology of its symbolic character in the construction of kinship, by questioning its position as the "natural" basis and unique factor in the creation of kinship (Biblarz & Stacey, 2010; Kroløkke et al., 2015). This does not mean that choice and will have taken the place of biology in the construction of kinship, but that we are witnessing a tension between biology and choice, in which, according to Stone (2013), choice is presented as a new "order". Making the relational aspect of kinship, the non-biological process of procreation, explicit and visible confronts individuals with an exercise in self-reflection and definition of family identity in which "the thickness of blood" is no longer fundamental. This does not mean that it does not continue to exert pressure on the representations and conceptions of kinship and family. Solo mothers by choice constitute an important case where that pressure is visible.

Studies on new family forms

The study of families produced through assisted reproduction is still sparse. Susan Golombok in the field of psychology in the United Kingdom and Maria Isabel Jociles-Rubio in the field of social anthropology in Spain were the most prolific authors in this area, according to a Scopus search carried out at the end of 2018. The purpose of this section is to critically analyze these authors' theoretical approaches and consider the elements necessary to developing a holistic and intersectional analysis that incorporates contemporary theorizations of new family forms and overcomes narrow biologistic outlooks. To that end it considers the questions, the analysis, and the interpretations of the studies conducted. In the case of the United Kingdom, Golombok's (1984) studies began in the 1980s in the context of the debates of the "Committee of Inquiry Into Human Fertilisation and Embryology". This was concerned with the possible negative impact of the new technologies of assisted reproduction on the functioning of families and the psychological development of the children, as well as with attitudes towards semen or egg donors and the parental bonding to children conceived via these techniques (Bolton et al., 1991).

The UK debates on assisted reproduction at the time included whether lesbian or heterosexual single women should be allowed access to assisted reproductive technologies, and specifically to sperm donation, to be able to conceive a child without the involvement of a man (Englert, 1994). Access to sperm donation had been denied to lesbian and single heterosexual women because it was argued that they could not provide a suitable family environment for children in that the children would have two mothers with no genetic connection to one of them. For lesbian as well as single heterosexual women, it was argued that the lack of a father could be detrimental, in that both the existence of an anonymous donor and the lack of a father might lead to psychosocial difficulties for the child. In response to such fears and assumptions, the research by Golombok and her co-authors were designed to compare biological nuclear families and families formed through assisted reproductive technologies.

Over the last three decades, evidence from their studies on the psychological development of the children of families formed by single heterosexual or lesbian mothers have failed to find empirical support to endorse the assumptions that (1) the children would show atypical development, (2) they would develop behavioral and emotional problems and difficulties in peer relations, and (3) the mothers would not be good mothers (Falk, 1989; Golombok & Tasker, 1994). Contrary to the concerns expressed in these debates, the results of Golombok's studies and of other research showed that "the quality of parenting in families with a child conceived by assisted conception is superior to that shown by families with a naturally conceived child" (Golombok et al., 1993, p. 17). No differences were found in the groups with respect to the emotions of the children, their behavior, or their relationships with their parents. Moreover, the consistent conclusion from these studies over the last 30 years is that the genetic bond is less important for family functioning than a strong desire to be parents by having children (Golombok, 2018; Golombok & Tasker, 1994). In the case of Spain, Law 14/2006 establishes that all women older than 18 years can be a beneficiary of assisted reproduction techniques regardless of their marital status and sexual orientation. Jociles-Rubio and and Rivas Rivas (2010) began to publish studies at the end of the first decade of this century on single mothers by choice, above all adoptive mothers and to a lesser degree single mothers who used assisted reproductive technologies. Her publications reproduced research questions similar to those posed by Golombok in the British context, such as the following: who become single mothers by choice (Jociles-Rubio et al., 2008), how families with children from gamete donation deal with the origins of their children (Jociles-Rubio et al., 2014), or the representation of kinship as a result of assisted reproductive techniques with a donor (Jociles-Rubio & Rivas-Rivas, 2016). Jociles also compares single mothers by choice in Spain and the United States (Hertz et al., 2016), showing that single mothers by choice in Spain are far more vocal and politically active than in the United States. However, Jociles's samples are limited because she draws her qualitative sample of single mothers by choice from associations such as Madres Solteras por Elección and their participation in the media, thus excluding "single" mothers by choice who do not belong to any association and who are not politically active. Another qualitative study undertaken in Spain reveals that half of the sample of solo women who have children through assisted reproduction are not politically active and, in addition, opt for a male chauvinist and Roman Catholic education for their children that will be analyzed in chapter 6.

Therefore, the families of solo mothers by choice are highly heterogeneous and should not be homogenized by forcing them to fit into a stereotype. As can be seen from the earlier discussion, the studies of Golombok and Jociles-Rubio orient to the same issues and begin with the same questions. Both focus on (a) comparing families that are formed through assisted reproduction or adoption with what might be considered "traditional biological nuclear families", (b) analyzing the adjustment of children in the new families (who "lack" genetic bonds) compared with "biological nuclear families", and (c) examining how the mothers and fathers of the new families reveal or do not reveal the information that their children were born thanks to assisted reproductive technologies, and the effect that the revelation can have on their offspring. These studies have helpfully shown that concerns about the children born from assisted reproduction or adopted children are misplaced. It would, therefore, seem timely to shift the focus of research away from comparing them with biological nuclear families. In her 2017 article, Golombok draws conclusions from her longitudinal study (started in 2000) on families formed through egg or sperm donation, and the consequences of assisted reproductive technologies on the development of their children. In her article, she asserts that, contrary to the concerns (she does not specify whose, perhaps the debates in the 1980s mentioned earlier), the new family compositions are characterized by positive parenting and well-adjusted children, because the children were very much wished and planned for. She goes on to state that, from a theoretical perspective, what this study tells us is that the number, gender, sexual orientation, and biological relation of the parents and children have less influence on the children's psychological development than the quality of the family relationships and the social context in which the children are raised, much the same conclusion that she reached in 1994 (Golombok & Tasker, 1994).

However, at no point does Golombok or Jociles-Rubio call into question the premise that the biological nuclear family as a structure and yardstick for other types of families. The question is whether there is a link between genetics and the well-being of the children. A wealth of research makes clear that this is not necessarily the case. For example, there are fathers, "deadbeat dads", who demonstrate that biological ties are no guarantee that fathers will ensure continuing investment of their resources in their own children (Dermott, 2008). Why, when Golombok and Jociles-Rubio discuss the structure of the hegemonic nuclear family, do they not delve deeper into its variety and explain the particularity of various structures? If the structure is formed by a father and a mother whose roles are unequal in a patriarchal family, how does this affect their children? Or when in a biological nuclear family the father is absent due to work or when both mother and father hire a succession of babysitters to look after their children because they both work until late, how do these circumstances affect their children (Li et al., 2014)? In their research, Golombok and Jociles-Rubio analyze the disclosure of the information regarding donors and the impact its concealment might have for children, presumably influenced by principles of good practice in adoption (Ghera, 2014; Morgan, 1999). However, they do not discuss the disclosure of other issues that are also important, that could affect children, but that are normally kept from them in biological nuclear families, such as infidelities, addictions, or toxic relations between family members. Similarly, Golombok and Jociles-Rubio do not mention the importance of other aspects such as managing injustices that lie at the heart of the hegemonic nuclear family. In particular, how does the lack of shared responsibilities between mothers and fathers with regard to the children, their care, and the household chores that has been repeatedly documented in both Spain and the United Kingdom (World Economic Forum, 2018) affect children in their upbringing and education? Furthermore, in the case of the United Kingdom, how does the fact that wealthy nuclear families send their children to boarding schools affect them? This is a phenomenon that has been called the "privileged abandonment" of children and that, according to Schaverien (2015), "Many adults are suffering long-term emotional or behavioral difficulties" (p. 84) – "boarding school syndrome" being recognized as a specific syndrome according to psychiatrists and psychologists. Strathern (1992) argues that new ideas are imagined through old ideas; what already exists may be set in common values and institutions and what people think is morally correct. Ideas are always put forward in contexts already occupied by other thoughts and images. Finding a place for new ideas becomes an act of displacement (Strathern, 1992).

For this reason, the concepts we employ to think other ideas are of importance. In this sense Golombok and Jociles-Rubio utilize old ideas to think about new phenomena. They pose old questions that are more suited to former eras to understand a new phenomenon that requires new questions and conceptualizations informed by the narratives and experiences of the women themselves who experience assisted reproduction without a partner. Families in Europe and the United States are more diverse than ever. However, the biological nuclear family still holds a strong symbolic significance and ideological relevance. Indeed, it is constructed as the gold standard of the family and the "best" environment for maternal and parental practices, particularly in the eyes of the creators of public policies and politicians. It has been argued that those who grow up in this type of family structure attain better academic results, experience less psychological distress, and less conflictual relationships with their parents, and who probably provided greater emotional support, cognitive stimulation, and supervision (Dunn et al., 1998; Goldberg, 2015; Neale, 2003; Setién, 2017). These assumptions, when combined with the ideology of the middle class of intensive parenting in the heterosexual nuclear family of two parents seen as ideal, ensure that mothering (from women who choose to become mothers on their own and who also work outside the home) is perceived as inferior, as there is no dedicated caregiver (aka mother) to provide full-time care to the child. As the rate of divorce began to increase in the West after 1945, and in the case of Spain from 1981 (due to the Franco dictatorship and the strong opposition of the Catholic Church, 45 years after the country's first divorce law, from 1932, was repealed), there have been many research studies on the impact of divorce on children. Two significant studies (Jenkins & Smith, 1993; Wallerstein & Blakeslee, 2002) found that divorce was often extremely difficult and disruptive to children and that the effects were long lasting. Their findings were influential on both public opinion and social policy in the United States, the United Kingdom, and beyond.

However, O'Connor et al. (2001) argued that this was not the case for all children and that while studies suggest that on average children progress in particular types of families, there are many children who progress in families that do not "fit" the norm, making the generalizations debatable. In fact, Mooney et al. (2009) in their report on the "Impact of Family Breakdown on Children's Well-Being. Evidence Review" conclude that "the majority of children will not be adversely affected in the long-term by family breakdown" (p. 3). How can we approach the subject from another angle? I believe the time has come to change the focus of attention of comparing families whose children have been born through assisted reproduction or adoption with biological nuclear families escaping the assumption that there is a link between genetics and the well-being of children. We need to interrogate the biological nuclear family as yardstick for other types of families, and we must reveal not only children's genetic origins but also all the information that may affect children's upbringing and psychological adjustment. New phenomena need different questions. To break new ground in understanding families produced through assisted technology, it is crucial to ask new questions and interrogate the very assumptions that have fueled research in the last two decades. DePaulo and Morris (2005) can help us to question one of the premises that Golombok and Jociles-Rubio use in their studies: the heterosexual biological family as the normative with which to compare other types of families. DePaulo (2014) explains that there exists in society a broad ideology that is neither contested nor recognized on marriage or couple cohabitation (and the biological nuclear family). Its premises are simply assumed, they are not questioned, perhaps because they offer a simple and satisfactory world view. DePaulo (2017) argues that when the number of adults not in a relationship was rising dramatically in the United States and Europe, academia was dominated by perspectives rooted in marriage or coupledom and in the nuclear family. It is undeniable that psychologists and other researchers who examine intrapersonal and interpersonal processes relevant to close relationships are inclined to studying dating relationships and marriages.

This is a research bias that has neglected singles and other meaningful close relationships (Clark & Graham, 2005). Nevertheless, those who come to research from other perspectives see that there are other questions to pose and other modes of analyzing and understanding these issues. According to DePaulo (2014), a singles studies perspective would bring to the field of interpersonal relationships a bigger, broader view of the people and relationships important to us in our lives. No longer would conjugal couples stand at the center of our relationship universes, with other adult relationship partners acting as the bit players orbiting around them (p. 66). Perspectives are needed that are anchored in the lives of "single" women, which represent people who have been marginalized for a long time or ignored in academic research. According to Reynolds and Wetherell (2003), academic research on singleness has largely assumed, if not quite pathology, at least that the psychology of the single woman will be shaped by "difference" and, possibly, personal "dysfunction".

Women in long-term relationships do not tend to be asked "how did you end up married?" Solo women, in contrast, are expected to explain her "condition", preferably a story of "circumstances" and "missed opportunities" or one that blames herself for being "unable to hold on to her man" (p. 492). Without "single" women's perspectives, academic research becomes narrow and suppositions are made that have not been adequately tested and that have an influence on the questions that are formulated, the data that are provided and how we interpret it. The diversity of experiences in the way that we live and think on the concept of family helps us to think about the world in modes that are not "too male, or too white or too married" (DePaulo, 2014) or too biological nuclear family. Reynolds and Wetherell (2003) and DePaulo and Morris (2005) argue that it is necessary to begin a conversation about single people and their place in society and in science. Both in society and in scientific texts, certain habitual ways of thinking have endured and remain implicit. In science, these habits have guided the type of questions that are posed, or the studies that are carried out, and how the results are interpreted. They have also shaped social interactions and public policies. The persistence of "singlism" (discrimination against single people, particularly against women) is manifested in the uncontested domination of the ideology of marriage or coupledom and the nuclear family (DePaulo, 2014). While sensitivity about diversity is more acute and it has become a commonplace that identities are multiple, including ethnicity, racialization, sex, gender, religion, social class, sexual orientation, age, and diverse capacities, that sensitivity does not extend to shifts in thinking about marital status, and the nuclear family which persist as key today. More than 30 years ago, Williams (1995) explained that:

> By the 1980s changing patterns of women's paid employment, especially within welfare states, changing household patterns particularly in relation to marriage and parenthood (increases in divorce and lone parenthood), an ageing population, increased female poverty, and the articulation of women's demands through women's movements have all challenged the relationship of the family to the needs, demands, and support for social policies.
>
> (p. 143)

According to DePaulo (2014), singlism endures, because the ideology of marriage or partnership and the nuclear family goes on and the welfare state continues to be predicated on it. The persistence of the ideology of the nuclear family is central in the world view of Global North societies, the heterosexual nuclear family as a site where racialized, religious, and patriarchal Western notions of gendered hierarchies have been naturalized and institutionalized to maintain hetero-patriarchal power. For those solo women who have chosen to be mothers, this ideology sustains the myth that in the heterosexual couple and the nuclear family there is a level of happiness and completeness that a woman alone cannot reach or understand and therefore, cannot offer to her children. Yanagisako and Delaney (1995) argued that:

> Gender definition and value have been inherent in the Western theory of procreation, but procreation is not just about the natural; it includes an ontological dimension. Because gender is at the heart of these socio-religious systems it is not surprising that issues of gender and procreation—marriage, family, birth control, abortion, sexuality, homosexuality, new reproductive technology—are at the centre of contemporary debates in our society, for new beliefs and practices challenge the entire cosmological order.
>
> (p. 9)

The ideologies of nuclear family personal responsibility are prepackaged understandings that normalize them and protect the institution from criticism. To forge productive understandings of new family forms, it is, therefore, important to disrupt the taken-for-granted normalization of biological nuclear families. One way in which this needs to be done is through interrogating the terms used to define women who mother outside nuclear families. Problematizing the terms "single" and "solo" (mothers by choice). I consider that the use of the expressions (a) "single" by choice, (b) "solo mum", or (c) "choice mum" is problematic because the term "single" is defined by its opposition to "married": the defining element continues to be that of marriage or couple cohabitation. Orbach and Eichenbaum (2014) and Eichenbaum and Orbach (1987) argue that it has been an assumed norm that women need a partner relationship with a man. This explains why, socially and culturally, it is expected that women should establish heterosexual relationships instead of celebrating their identities as autonomous and independent.

Orbach and Eichenbaum indicate that the women in their psychotherapy center admit that they stay in unsatisfactory relationships for fear of losing themselves. They suggest that women think that their identity is constructed in a partner relationship and for that reason, they seek a relationship not only to connect with someone but also to construct their own identity. The term "solo" (mums) is a Spanish usage that refers to being "alone; without family or friends". This entails a falsehood in the case of the majority of women who decide to have children on their own, as in general they have family and friends that support them. The expression of "choice" (mums) alludes to the conscious choice to have children, but does not include the fact of choosing to be mothers without the involvement of a partner. Those women who are in a relationship can also choose whether or not to become mothers. Each of the three expressions discussed previously present difficulties when it comes to defining this group of women who have decided to have children on their own. Creating categories through language means labelling experiences, yet the categories come into being with attendant social power relations that exist in the sociocultural context concerned. They are not neutral, but can serve to recreate relations of dominance and subordination that are reflected in dominant discourses (May, 2006), influencing the ways in which we perceive those groups and how they can feel about themselves (Taylor & Bogdan, 1998). By defining women by their lack of a relationship with a man, the categories of "single" or "solo" may reproduce the hegemonic viewpoint of mothers and families. These women's transition to motherhood on their own has, according to them, brought about an experience of empowerment and emancipation, enabling them to fulfil their wishes to be mothers and to provide their children with positive models of motherhood enacting their reproductive agency. Therefore, a different term is necessary, one that recognizes this group of women as autonomous and independent, living differently the normative forms of procreative life.

Research findings

It is key at this point to empirically create new insights and knowledge setting up a dialogue between (a) the persistence of the comparative focus on the nuclear biological family, new forms of family, and the children's well-being, in the publications of Golombok, Jociles, and their co-authors analyzed in previous sections, and (b) the analysis of the findings of my ethnographic fieldwork in Spain and in the United Kingdom as well as the examination of a child's drawing on her family, which will be discussed in the next section. This dialogue is relevant as some of the findings contrast with the conclusions reached by the studies explored in previous sections. Before choosing to become mothers, the interviewees in this study have already made a decision as to the emotional, psychological, and social irrelevance of the genetic material. Genetics is important regarding the heredity of diseases, in the same way as it is for other families in society: none want their children to get inherited diseases that will condition their lives. However, genetics loses symbolic relevance in the face of their persistent desire to be a mother (regardless of their national, ethnic, religious origin, or social class). Depending on the case, for the women I interviewed, being a mother has involved sperm, egg, or embryo donation; in one case seven cycles of assisted reproduction and for some of them years of failed attempts, and in other cases they suffered numerous miscarriages. For this reason, genetics and disclosure are not at the top of their list of priorities as one might think reading some of the scientific literature or some of the media coverage on this subject. All the women interviewed for this study started explaining to their children how they were conceived since they were babies with story books that dealt with their specific form of family. In fact, some of the participants made their own story books with their own words and pictures of their children. Participants in both countries demonstrate a broad knowledge of assisted reproductive technologies and different reproductive national laws. They know where to find (non) anonymous donors, have read the latest research on epigenetics, and have engaged in physical and virtual forums, networks, and associations specialized in becoming a "solo" mother. Jen and Toni are two examples that epitomize this. Jen, one of the participants, a Londoner who arrived from Poland in the 1990s flew to a clinic in Spain to become pregnant with her child from an anonymous double donation at the age of 45. She explains how she gathered information years before deciding to become pregnant:

> I went several times to a big fertility show which runs in November every year in Olympia, attended lots of seminars where fertility experts and clinics shared

> the latest research, there were also women who shared their personal experience. I started researching about epigenetics which really inspired me.

Toni, a 42-year-old Spaniard living in Andalusia explained how she arrived at the decision of becoming pregnant with the help of an anonymous sperm donor in a clinic in Spain:

> First I got all the information I could for a year, I read a lot, visited many specialised websites and clinics. I ended up writing 5 pages of questions to which I expected answers from each clinic I visited. At the end I chose the clinic not only for their success rates, treatment and price, but also for the human team behind it.

Their handling and knowledge of the reproductive technologies as well as their preparation for making the decision puts them in a privileged position in that they have consulted specialist literature and visited websites where genetics and epigenetics are explained, and where experiences of the different phases of the process of becoming a mother by choice are: thinking about the decision to become a mother, trying to get pregnant, failing in the attempts, going through the first phases of pregnancy, becoming a mother of a baby through donation, visiting various assisted reproduction clinics. These women have researched what the reproductive technology market has to offer on a national and international level. Nineteen of the 30 women interviewed in London had been treated in clinics or had obtained genetic material in Spain, Greece, Denmark, or the United States. When I attended a 1-day workshop in London run by a charity dealing with issues on assisted reproductive technologies and disclosure to their children, out of 13 cases 54% of that sample (7) were treated in Spain, 38% in the United Kingdom (5), and 7% (1) somewhere else in Europe; 8 were white British heterosexual couples, 1 was a white American lesbian couple, and there were 4 solo mothers by choice (2 from Britain and 2 from European countries). Therefore, their knowledge places them in an advantageous position when it comes to thinking about genetics and whether it is relevant or not in their lives with their children.

This does not mean dismissing the importance of the genetic conditions that may affect their children, or that social issues may arise for the children, but it has nothing to do with relating biology or genetics with kinship or the family, dismissing the assumption that family is only a family if there's a genetic link between the parents and the child. These women also decided that they had sufficient economic resources and the appropriate social networks for when the baby arrived. This means that they have already thought strategically about all these issues before their pregnancy and they accept the consequences of what it involves, including how best to deal in an age-appropriate way with all their children's queries, as well as thinking beforehand about the possible questions arising in their family, work, and social settings. How do children think of "family"? The phrase "blood is thicker than water" in Europe and the United States suggests that biological relations are fundamental to how the idea of family is conceived. However, for most children in these places, genetics holds little significance, especially before the age of five, as the psychologist Jean Piaget (1929) discovered. He studied the ideas about family given by children of different ages and found that, before the age of five, children saw the family simply as the people who lived with them and did not talk of kinship. More recent anthropological and sociological research suggests that this is still the case: the idea of biological relatives only begins to be important for children over the age of eight (Christensen & James, 2017; Cooper et al., 2018; Zvara et al., 2014), although depending on the sociocultural and religious environment the emphasis on biology can vary, as, for example, in the case of the Jewish community. Jewish children were found to be particularly aware of their biological relatedness, reflecting a specific world view of the religious relation with genetics, the basic belief of which is the transmission of Jewish identity through genetic heredity from the mother (Blake et al., 2013; Roe et al., 2006). In the case of two Jewish participants, Sonia who is a 43-year-old woman, originally from Europe and resident in London, did not wish to reveal to her synagogue and the rabbi that her child was the result of egg donation, as well as sperm donation, because the egg donor was not Jewish. Sonia had migrated to London more than 20 years previously, while her family remained in her country of origin, and therefore she felt that she only needed to give explanations to those in her most immediate surroundings: to her acquaintances, her synagogue, and her rabbi; but she had decided to conceal the information that her baby did not possess her genes for fear that her child would be excluded from Jewish identity in her religious community.

The other participant, Claire, 63 years old, Jewish, who was born in a former British colony and who migrated to London 40 years ago, has a 23-year-old son who was conceived with the sperm from a Jewish donor. She claimed it was important to her that the donor was Jewish even though the Code of Jewish Law states that a child of a Jewish mother is Jewish, regardless of the father's lineage (Posner, 2019). Therefore these mothers' views may influence the importance that their children attribute to genetics in relation to their Jew identity. Does the importance children give to genetics depend on the world view of the mothers/fathers and their family and friendship environments? In the case of the Jewish community, the fact that a child is the result of egg donation from a non-Jewish donor can mean exclusion from their religious community, but if genetics lacked importance, would it be relevant for the child? Carol Smart (2002, 2003) and her colleagues carried out three qualitative research projects in the United Kingdom that involved speaking with children about their families after divorce to analyze how their views developed and changed. The first study entailed in-depth interviews with 52 children, most of them aged between 7 and 14 years, from a wide range of socioeconomic backgrounds. The majority were living with one parent and seeing the other at weekends. In the second study, they interviewed 65 children who were being "coparented' (spending equal amounts of time with both parents, after divorce or separation). She argues that genetics do not matter to children, what matters to them is that in their homes the adults provide them with love and security, and that it is the quality of family relationships and the provision of emotional and material security that has a much more significant meaning for children than the structure of the home, the gender, or the number of adults that it contains. Smart (2002) and her colleagues identified three aspects of family relations that the children valued and that take on different meanings depending on their age: (a) residence, who lives where and with whom, which is particularly important for children up until 7 or 8 years old; (b) the family roles, what the family members do for one another, a debate that is a concern for 8- to 12-year-olds; and (c) the quality of these relations: the love, care, and respect that the children perceive within the home, being important issues for children. Smart (2002) and Tipper (2011) who analyzed children's own perspectives on their connections with animals conclude that, in many senses, children are more flexible than adults about what constitutes the family and they include a large number of people in their description of their families, as living and dead relatives and members of other households, including pets. This is epitomized by an example of the study I conducted: the drawing made by Vera (Figure 2.1), the 6-year-old daughter of 51-year-old Paula, a Spaniard who conceived Vera with the help of anonymous egg and sperm donors in a clinic in Spain. At school they asked Vera to draw her family, and she did so, thus.

Starting from the left-hand side: (a) her godmother (her grandmother's friend) auntie Julia; (b) her godfather, whom she calls uncle Antonio (married to Julia, and a friend of her grandparents); (c) Juan, her cousin (12 years old at the time); (d) Pedro, her cousin, Juan's brother (14 years old at the time); (e) Vera, 6 years old; (f) Bimba, her cousins' dog; (g) her aunt (her mum's sister who is Pedro and Juan's mother); (h) her mother; (i) her grandmother (her mother's mother); (j) her grandfather (her mother's father) who died when Vera was 2 years old, Vera drew him in a coffin with a cross on top; and (k) her great-grandmother (her mother's

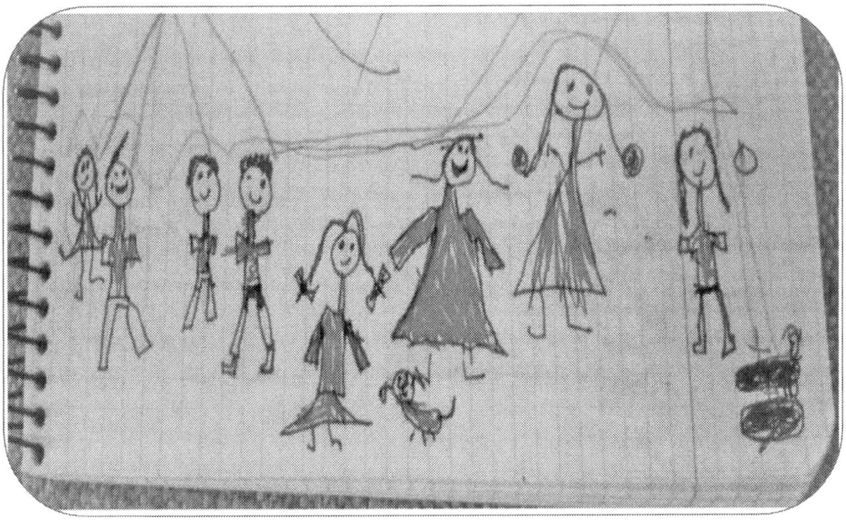

Figure 2.1 Illustration drawn by Vera; photograph taken by author.

grandmother) who died 27 years before Vera was born. She also drew her in a coffin with a cross on top. Hence for Vera, her cousins' dog and her great-grandmother who died many years before she was born, or her grandfather whom she can't remember because he died when she was a toddler, are all part of her family: human beings and a pet that, in Vera's imaginary of affective relationships, are meaningful. Kaplan and Main (1986) found that drawings by children with secure attachment were realistic; figures were complete, grounded, and individuated, not drawn exactly alike. There was also a natural proximity between family members and an impression of happiness in the family. Zvara et al. (2014) state "that children's drawings are a window into the way they view their home life". In their study, in which 962 first-graders (6- and 7-year-olds) participated, the children were asked to draw their families, and those children from "high-functioning" homes represented the members of their families with appropriate differentiation, for example, with the parents drawn larger than the children.

Blake et al. (2013) and her team have also studied children born in a variety of family structures – including solo mothers by choice and same-sex couples – and they concluded that children younger than 7 years old showed little comprehension about what egg or sperm donation means. By the age of 10, they can understand the non-genetic heredity of their mother(s) and/or father(s), and their reactions varied between indifference and curiosity. In another study, Golombok et al. (2016) compared 51 families of solo mothers by choice with 52 biparental families, all with children between the ages of 4 and 9 years, conceived by the donation of genetic material, and analyzed the psychological adjustment of the children of single mothers by choice, comparing this with families of divorced and separated families, with families in poverty, and with families whose parents suffer from depression. The only difference, they conclude, in parenting quality between these types of family is that there are fewer conflicts between mother and child in the solo-mother-by-choice families. The perceived economic difficulties, the gender of the child, or parental stress was associated with the children's adjustment problems in both types of family. The results of this study suggest that solo motherhood by choice, in itself, does not cause psychological problems for the children. Years ago Golombok and Tasker (1994) had arrived at the same conclusion:

> The finding that the quality of parenting in heterosexual families created as a result of assisted reproduction is particularly good and that the children are functioning well suggests that the use of donor insemination by lesbian or single heterosexual women would not, in itself, lead to difficulties for the children.
>
> (p. 1975)

Nonetheless, Golombok et al. (2016) do declare that "the single mothers showed lower levels of interaction and sensitivity responding to their infants than did the married mothers" (p. 410), without explaining how they reached this conclusion, and indicating that it was "possibly because the presence of a partner allowed the married mothers more time with their babies" (p. 410). However, the authors do not support this assertion with interview quotations or observations from fieldwork. On the other hand, they state that although the mothers of both family types showed positive relationships with their children, the single mothers showed greater joy and less anger towards their children, according to the Parent Development Interview, an interview technique designed to evaluate the nature of the emotional bond between mother and child (Slade, Belsky, Aber & Phelps, 1999, cited in Golombok et al., 2016). Despite the fact that applying a 1999 methodological tool in the current context may be inappropriate, Golombok et al. (2016) do not specify what is understood by "emotional bond" and how it is expressed. It certainly varies over the first 12 years of life. Cooper et al. (2018) argue that motherhood and fatherhood change over time and over the lives of individuals: "the same person who has two children will be a very different parent to the first child than to the second" (p. 8). Therefore, I understand that the same mother may show different emotional bonds with her children, and that emotional bonds also may change over time. Third, the emotional bond would vary depending on the sociocultural, historical, religious, and economic context. Weinraub, Horvath, and Gringlas suggest that single-parent families that arise from different circumstances differ in a number of important ways, and that these differences must be considered for understanding of the more general effects of rearing children in a single-parent family. "One of the most important characteristics of single-parent families and their children is their heterogeneity" (Weinraub et al., 2002, p. 110). However, Golombok et al. do not take these aspects and variations into account as limitations of the methodological tool that they use and therefore as limitations of their study.

Reflections: a new research agenda

The aim of this chapter was to compare and contrast the findings of the ethnographic study that I conducted in Spain and the United Kingdom and a meta-ethnography, in which studies on "single" mothers by choice from the most prolific scholars, according to Scopus (2018), were examined to produce new understandings and knowledge. First, the terms of "single" and "solo" mothers by choice found in the literature as categories for women who chose to become mothers on their own have been critiqued, as those adjectives may reproduce the hegemonic viewpoint of defining women by their lack of a relationship with a man. This treatment denies women's autonomy and self-determination. Furthermore, the terms "single" and "solo" do not represent the experiences of the majority of women interviewed for whom family, friends, social networks, and community groups are important. Second, the premises found in the literature on the conceptualization of the relationship between the social and the biological in societies of the Global North on new forms of family persistently persevere on the comparative focus between the biological nuclear family and new forms of family. My argument is that this is controversial because (a) we need to call into question the premise of the biological nuclear family as a yardstick for other types of families and (b) it essentializes diverse types of families, silencing differences within the categories. The question thus arises of why one type of family – donor-conceived families and adoptive families – is routinely compared with another type of family – the biological nuclear –without raising questions about the variety and complexity of each type of family in work by, for example, Golombok, Jociles-Rubio, their co-authors, and other scholars. Consequently, how can the family diversity within each of the categories the authors study affect children? I consider that those authors strip the families in their studies of complexity, reducing and simplifying their difference to one element: the lack of genetic relation between mothers, fathers, and children erroneously linking genetics with kinship or the family. Third, Golombok and Jociles-Rubio repeatedly focus on the children's adjustment in donor-conceived families as if there was a relation between genetics and the well-being of the children, instead of taking on board research studies examined in previous sections that conclude that what matters to children is not genetics, the structure of the home, or the gender of their parents, but that adults in their homes provide them with love and security.

As discussed in the findings, for the women interviewed genetics were only relevant regarding the heredity of diseases, but lost symbolic importance when participants faced their deep desire to become mothers. Moreover, children's drawings show the irrelevance of genetics; pictures include alive and deceased human beings and pets that form their imaginary of affective relationships. Geneticist biologist Prof. Kornblihtt (2018) claims that there is a tendency to exaggerate the role of genes and underestimate the role of the environment, culture, and society; he stresses that genetic identity is not the same as human identity. Furthermore, Lipton (2015), a cell biologist, underlines the importance of epigenetics, how the environment including nutrition, stress, and emotions can modify the donors' genes in the woman's womb without changing the basic blueprint. Likewise, James (2016), a clinical child psychologist, emphasizes that "the myth that we are carcasses for reproducing our genes should be replaced with the fact that traits are passed down through patterns of nurture" (p. 212). Therefore, situating the issue in the genes of the child displaces the focus away from the society that created that family, in particular, in societies of the Global North where the hetero-normative construction of "family" in biological nuclear terms is embedded in patriarchal, religious, and racialized power relations, and therefore must not be taken for granted as a concept. Neither of the authors (Golombok and Jociles-Rubio) adopts an intersectional methodological perspective (Collins, 2000) that recognizes that all families, regardless of their genetic makeup, are formed through different positions and different structures – singlism, ageism, heterosexism, sexual orientation, social class, ability, racialization, ethnicity, religious beliefs – and that, consequently, the effects of these intersections may influence families and their children's experiences.

The theories of intersectionality are useful in this case because they argue that social structures are complex and interact between one another (Browne & Misra, 2003; Crenshaw, 1991; May, 2006). There is no uniform structure in which the individuals of the same social class or the same ethnic background live. Rather, each individual inhabits a multitude of structures that intersect. For example, compare two cases taken from my fieldwork in London: Rose, white British, lives in London and used a non-anonymous sperm donor from a US sperm bank. She earns £100,000 a year, pays £1,500 a month for her child's nursery school, and has a network of babysitters, family, and friends that supports her. Tania, on the other hand, is a European Jew who arrived in London in the 1990s; she used anonymous egg and sperm donors from a clinic in Spain and was concerned about her egg donor being non-Jew. She is a key worker with a salary of £28,000 a year and has to depend on the city council for housing, her family of origin is abroad, and her friendship network is limited. The only category these participants share is that of women who decided to have donor-conceived children on their own. Some of the social structures they occupy could lead to discrimination or vulnerability, such as not being British in the United Kingdom (especially after Brexit), being a key worker (low salary), and dependent on council housing, or having meager support networks. Other structures can represent social privilege: being white British in the United Kingdom, belonging to the middle class, and enjoying several support networks. We also need to consider (a) the differences in laws on assisted reproduction that are constrained by elements such as accessibility and affordability, and moral approval or rejection of society, and (b) the (non)anonymity of gamete donors in different countries and how those factors may impact donor-conceived families. Therefore, these structures are intersected and cannot be reduced to each of the categories that form them. In other words, the analyses presented by Golombok and Jociles-Rubio reduce the categories of singlehood and, in this case, the biological nuclear family to one-dimensional categories. Finally, there is a need to study families as intersections of diverse social structures, as loci of power relations, and as processes which take place inside individuals that belong to culturally embedded groups. The intersection of all those positions are important to analysis, as are different reproductive politics, affordable and good-quality child care services that contribute to child development, gender, and socioeconomic equity.

References

Biblarz, T. J., & Stacey, J. (2010). How does the gender of parents matter? *Journal of Marriage and Family, 72*(1), 3–22.

Blake, L., Casey, P., Jadva, V., & Golombok, S. (2013). "I was quite amazed": Donor conception and parent-child relationships from the child's perspective. *Children and Society, 28*(6), 425–437. https://doi.org/10.1111/chso.12014

Bolton, V., Golombok, S., Cook, R., Bish, A., & Rust, J. (1991). A comparative study of attitudes towards donor insemination and egg donation in recipients' potential donors and the public. *Journal of Psychosomatic Obstetrics & Gynecology, 12*(3), 217–228. https://doi.org/10.3109/01674829109078003

Browne, I., & Misra, J. (2003). The intersection of gender and race in the labour market. *Annual Review of Sociology, 29*, 487–513.

Carsten, J. (2000). Introduction: Cultures of relatedness. In J. Carsten (Ed.), *Cultures of relatedness: New approaches to the study of kinship*. London: Cambridge University Press.

Chodorow, N. (1978). *The reproduction of mothering*. Berkeley, CA: University of California Press.

Christensen, P., & James, A. (Eds.). (2017). *Research with children: Perspectives and practices*. Oxon: Routledge.
Clark, M. S., & Graham, S. M. (2005). Do relationship researchers neglect singles? Can we do better? *Psychological Inquiry, 16*(2–3), 131–136.
Collins, P. H. (2000). *Black feminist thought: Knowledge, consciousness, and the politics of empowerment*. New York: Routledge.
Cooper, V. L., Montgomery, H., & Kieron, S. (2018). *Parenting the first twelve years: What evidence tells us*. Cape Town: Pelican Books.
Crenshaw, K. (1991). Mapping the margins: Intersectionality, identity politics and violence against women of color. *Standfored Law Review, 43*(6), 1241–1299.
Daniels, K. (2006). *Building a family with the assistance of donor insemination*. Auckland: Dunmore Publishers.
DePaulo, B. (2014). A singles studies perspective on mount marriage. *Psychological Inquiry, 25*(1), 64–68. https://doi.org/10.1080/1047840X.2014.878173
DePaulo, B. (2017). The urgent need for a singles studies discipline. *Signs: Journal of Women in Culture and Society, 42*(4), 1015–1019. https://doi.org/10.1086/690956
DePaulo, B. M., & Morris, W. L. (2005). Singles in society and in science. *Psychological Inquiry, 16*(2–3), 57–83. https://doi.org/10.1207/s15327965pli162&3_01
Dermott, E. (2008). Paradoxes of contemporary fatherhood. In E. Dermott (Ed.), *Intimate fatherhood: A sociological analysis* (pp. 7–24). London: Routledge.
Dunn, J., Deater-Deckard, K., Pickering, K., & O'Connor, T. G. (1998). Children adjustment and pro-social behaviour in step, single parent, and non-stepfamily settings: Findings from a community study. *Journal of Child Psychology and Psychiatry, 39*(8), 1083–1095. https://doi.org/10.1111/1469-7610.00413
Eichenbaum, L., & Orbach, S. (1987). Separation and intimacy: Crucial practice issues in working with women in therapy. In S. Ernst & M. Maguire (Eds.), *Living with the sphinx: Papers from the women's therapy centre* (pp. 49–67). London: Women's Press.
Englert, Y. (1994). Artificial insemination of single and lesbian women with donor semen. *Human Reproduction, 9*(11), 1969–1971. https://doi.org/10.1093/oxfordjournals.humrep.a138372
Falk, P. J. (1989). Lesbian mothers: Psychosocial assumptions in family law. *American Psychologist, 44*(6), 941–947.
Ghera, M. (2014). Past adoption practices and the disclosure of adoption information. http://researchbriefings.files.parliament.uk/documents/SN06379/SN06379.pdf
Glenn, E., Chang, G., & Forcey, L. R. (Eds.). (1994). *Mothering: Ideology, experience, and agency*. New York: Routledge.
Goldberg, J. (2015). Why family matters, and why traditional families are still best. www.latimes.com/opinion/op-ed/la-oe1027-goldberg-family-structure-20151027-column.html
Golombok, S. (1984) Children in lesbian and single parent lesbian households. Proceedings of Boerhaave Conference on Child and Adolescent Psychiatry, Leiden, 1984. IP-Gegevens Koninklijke Bibliotheek, The Hague.
Golombok, S. (2018). Research on assisted reproduction families: A historical perspective. In G. Kovacs, P. Brinsden, & A. DeCherney (Eds.), *In vitro fertilization and assisted reproduction: A history* (pp. 240–247). Cambridge: Cambridge University Press.
Golombok, S., Cook, R., Bish, A., & Murray, C. (1993). Quality of parenting in families created by the new reproductive technologies: A brief report of preliminary findings. *Journal of Psychosomatic Obstetrics and Gynaecology, 14*, 17–22.

Golombok, S., & Tasker, F. (1994). Donor insemination for single heterosexual and lesbian women: Issues concerning the welfare of the child. *Human Reproduction, 11*(9), 1972–1976.

Golombok, S., Zadeh, S., Imrie, S., Smith, V., & Freeman, T. (2016). Single mothers by choice: Mother–child relationships and children's psychological adjustment. *Journal of Family Psychology, 30*, 409–418. https://doi.org/10.1037/fam0000188

Hertz, R., Rivas, A. M., & Rubio Jociles, M. I. (2016). Single mothers by choice in Spain and the United States. In C. L. Shehan (Ed.), *Encyclopedia of family studies* (pp. 1–5). Hoboken, NJ: Wiley Blackwell.

James, O. (2016). *Not in your genes: The real reasons children are like their parents*. New York: Penguin Random House.

Jenkins, J. M., & Smith, M. A. (1993). A prospective study of behavioural disturbance in children who subsequently experience parental divorce. *Journal of Divorce & Remarriage, 19*(1–2), 143–160. https://doi.org/10.1300/J087v19n01_08

Jociles Rubio, M. I. and Rivas Rivas, A. M. (2010). Es la ausencia del padre un problema? La disociación de los roles paternos entre las madres solteras por elección. *Gazeta de antropología, 26*(1), 4. www.gazeta-antropologia.es/?p=1547

Jociles-Rubio, M. I., & Rivas-Rivas, A. M. (2016). Cambios en la concepción y representación del parentesco a raíz del uso de las técnicas de reproducción asistida con donante [Changes in the conception and representation of kinship due to the use of assisted reproductive technologies with donors]. Ankulegi. *Revista de Antropología* [*Journal of Anthropology*], *20*, 63–78.

Jociles-Rubio, M. I., Rivas-Rivas, A., Moncó, B., Villamil, F., & Díaz, P. (2008). Una reflexión crítica sobre la monoparentalidad: El caso de las madres solteras por elección [A critical reflection on single parenthood: The case of single mothers by choice]. Portularia. *Revista de Trabajo Social* [*Journal of Social Work*], *VIII*, 265–274.

Jociles-Rubio, M. I., Rivas-Rivas, A. M., & Poveda-Bicknell, D. (2014). Monoparentalidad por elección y revelación de los orígenes a los hijos nacidos por donación de gametos [Single parents by choice and disclosure of origins to children born from donation of gametes]. El caso de España [The case of Spain]. Retrieved from www.scielo.org.mx/scielo.php?script=sci_ abstract&pid=S1405-14352014000200003&lng=pt&nrm=iso

Kaplan, N., & Main, M. (1986). *Instructions for the classification of children's family drawings in terms of representation of attachment*. Berkeley, CA: University of California.

Kornblihtt, A. (2018). *Un embrión no es lo mismo que un ser humano*. Pleanario IVE. Retrieved from www.laizquierdadiario.com/AlbertoKornblihtt-Un-embrion-no-es-lo-mismo-que-un-ser-humano

Kroløkke, C., Myong, L., Adrian, S. W., & Tjørnhøj-Thomsen, T. (Eds.). (2015). *Critical kinship studies*. Lanham, MD: Rowman & Littlefield.

Lamphere, L. (2001). Whatever happened to kinship studies? Reflections of a feminist anthropologist. In L. Stone (Ed.), *New directions in anthropological kinship*. Lanham, MD: Rowman & Littlefield Publishers.

Li, J., Johnson, S. E., Han, W. J., Andrews, S., Kendall, G., Strazdins, L., & Dockery, A. (2014). Parents' nonstandard work schedules and child well-being: A critical review of the literature. *The Journal of Primary Prevention, 35*(1), 53–73. https://doi.org/10.1007/s10935-013-0318-z

Lipton, B. H. (2015). *The biology of belief*. London: Hay House.

May, V. (2006). Lone motherhoods in context (ESRC National Centre for Research Methods). NCRM Working Paper Series 5/06. University of Manchester. Retrieved from https://pdfs.semanticscholar.org/114f/9b5c7394156a7871d4bd1421d5e7d8960a32.pdf

Mooney, A., Oliver, C., & Smith, M. (2009). Impact of family breakdown on children's well-being evidence. Retrieved from https://dera.ioe.ac.uk/11165/1/DCSF-RR113.pdf

Morgan, P. (1999). *Adoption: The continuing debate*. London: IEA Health and Welfare Unit.

Neale, J. (2003). *Citizenship for children: Strategies for development*. York: Joseph Rowntree Foundation.

O'Connor, T. G., Dunn, J., Jenkins, J. M., Pickering, K., & Rabasj, J. (2001). Family settings and children's adjustment within and across families. *British Journal of Psychiatry, 179*(2), 110–115. https://doi.org/10.1192/bjp.179.2.110

Odeh, L. (2010). A comparative analysis of Global North and Global South economies. *Journal of Sustainable Development in Africa, 12*(3), 338–348.

Okin, S. (1989). *Justice, gender and the family*. New York: Basic Books.

Orbach, S., & Eichenbaum, L. (2014). *What do women want?* Scotts Valley, CA: CreateSpace Independent Publishing Platform.

O'Reilly, A. (Ed.). (2007). *Maternal theory: Essential readings*. Ontario: Demeter Press.

Phoenix, A., Woollett, A., & Lloyd, E. (Eds.). (1991). *Motherhood: Meanings, practices and ideologies*. Newcastle upon Tyne: Sage.

Piaget, J. (1929). *El juicio y el razonamiento en el niño*. Madrid: Ediciones La Lectura.

Posner, M. (2019). How do I know if I am a Jew? Retrieved from www.chabad.org/library/article_cdo/aid/3408865/jewish/How-Do-I-Know-If-I-Am-a-Jew.htm

Ragoné, H. (1994). *Surrogate motherhood: Conception in the heart*. Boulder, CO: Westview Press.

Reynolds, J., & Wetherell, M. (2003). The discursive climate of singleness: The consequences for women's negotiation of a single identity. *Feminism & Psychology, 13*(4), 489–510. https://doi.org/10.1177/09593535030134014

Rich, A. (1995). *Of woman born: Motherhood as experience and institution*. New York: W. W. Norton & Company.

Roe, A., Bridges, L., Dunn, J., & O'Connor, T. G. (2006). Young children's representations of their families: A longitudinal follow up study of family drawings by children living in different family settings. *International Journal of Behavioural Development, 30*(6), 529–536. doi.org/10.1177/0165025406072898

Schaverien, J. (2015). *Boarding school syndrome: The psychological trauma of the "privileged" child*. London: Routledge.

Schneider, D. M. (1980). *American kinship: A cultural account*. Chicago, IL: The University of Chicago Press.

Schneider, D. M. (1984). *A critique of the study of kinship*. Ann Arbor, MI: The University of Michigan.

Setién, M. (2017). El modelo de familia clásico es el más beneficioso para los niños [The classic family model is the most beneficial for children]. *ABC*. Retrieved from www.abc.es/familia/padres-hijos/ abci-modelo-familia-clasico-mas-beneficioso-para-ninos-201703091558_noticia.html

Slade, A., Belsky, J., Aber, J. L., & Phelps, J. L. (1999). Mothers' representations of their relationships with their toddlers: Links to adult attachment and observed mothering. *Developmental Psychology, 35*(3), 611–619. https://doi.org/10.1037/0012-1649.35.3.611

Smart, C. (2002). From children's shoes to children's voices. *Family Court Review, 40*(3), 307–319. www.naccc.org.uk/downloads/Childrens_shoes_to_childrens_voices. Pdf

Smart, C. (2003). Introduction: New perspectives on childhood and divorce. *Childhood, 10*(2), 123–129. https://doi.org/10.1177/0907568203010002001

Stone, L. (Ed.). (2001). *New directions in anthropological kinship*. Lanham, MD: Rowman & Littlefield Publishers.

Stone, L. (2013). *Kinship and gender*. Boulder, CO: Westview Press.

Strathern, M. (1992). *Reproducing the future: Anthropology, kinship and the new reproductive technologies*. London: Routledge.

Strauss, A., & Corbin, J. (1998). *Basics of qualitative research: Techniques and procedures for developing grounded theory*. Thousand Oaks, CA: Sage.

Taylor, S. J., & Bogdan, R. (1998). *Introduction to qualitative research methods: A guidebook and resource* (3rd ed.). Hoboken, NJ: John Wiley & Sons Inc.

Tipper, B. (2011). 'A dog who I know quite well': Everyday relationships between children and animals. *Children's Geographies, 9*(2), 145–165. https://doi.org/10.1080/147332 85.2011.562378

Wallerstein, J., & Blakeslee, S. (2002). *The unexpected legacy of divorce: A 25 year landmark study*. Westport, CT: Hyperion

Weinraub, M., Horvath, D. L., & Gringlas, M. B. (2002). Single parenthood. In M. H. Bornstein (Ed.), *Handbook of parenting: Being and becoming a parent* (pp. 109–140). Hillsdale, NJ: Lawrence Erlbaum Associates.

Williams, F. (1995). Race/ethnicity, gender, and class in welfare states: A framework for comparative analysis. *Social Politics: International Studies in Gender, State & Society, 2*(2), 127–159. https://doi.org/10.1093/sp/2.2.127

World Economic Forum. (2018). The global gender gap report. Retrieved from www3.weforum.org/docs/WEF_GGGR_2018.pdf

Yanagisako, S., & Delaney, C. (Eds.). (1995). *Naturalising power: Essays in feminist cultural analysis*. London: Routledge.

Zvara, B. J., Mills-Koonce, W. R., Garrett-Peters, P., Wagner, N. J., Vernon-Feagans, L., & Cox, M. (2014). The mediating role of parenting in the associations between household chaos and children's representations of family dysfunction. *Attachment & Human Development, 16*, 633–655. https://doi.org/10.1080/14 616734.2014.966124

3 Science, profits, and success rates

What about patient care?

This chapter is divided into four parts: the first will contextualize the economics of reproductive treatments; the second will explore the marketing strategies that clinics use; the third will examine consumer law, national commissions, personal gain, and ethical standards; and the last part will analyze participants' experiences.

The fertility business

The use of assisted reproductive technologies is increasing in the international context, not only by providing treatments to heterosexual couples with infertility problems, but also to solo individuals and same-sex couples who wish to have children (Kuhnt & Passet-Wittig, 2022). Worldwide, over 10 million babies have been born following ART procedures since 1978 (ESHRE, 2020). Europe leads the world in ART, initiating approximately 50% of all reported treatment cycles. Most ART treatments take place in women aged between 30 and 39 years. Not every treatment cycle, with all its challenges for patients and doctors, produces a baby. In Europe, the mean pregnancy rate per embryo transfer was 39% after in vitro fertilization (IVF), 40.2% after intracytoplasmic sperm injection (ICSI), 33.1% after frozen embryo transfer, and 49.2% after egg donation in 2017 (ESHRE, 2020). Many countries prohibit fertility treatment. As a result, such people travel abroad to countries where the legal framework, relevant to assisted reproduction and to becoming a parent, is favorable, growing into a key sector for investors looking to generate stronger profits from the largely stable medical or medical-technology sectors (Karadima, 2022). According to market analysts, providers of reproductive treatments reported profits of $12.5 billion in 2018, and are expected to generate profits of up to $25.6 billion in 2026 (Allied Market Research, 2021).

This predicted increase in profits in the coming years clearly shows that there is a large and highly profitable market for fertility treatments. A global reproductive economy already exists (Kossoudji, 2005). Crawford and Ledger (2019) argue that there are no signs that the market for ART is about to become saturated. Instead, new markets are opening up. With the ART market increasing in size steadily over the past few years, myriad opportunities have emerged for foreign investors to back projects in this area. Data from Pitchbook shows that $823.1m was invested across

DOI: 10.4324/9781003269755-4

90 deals globally in fertility technology venture capital in 2021, up from $132.2m and 18 deals in 2012 (Hodgson, 2022). Investments in fertility technology include projects related to egg freezing, machine learning for embryo selection, artificial wombs for premature babies, sperm count, IVF improvements, and diagnostic apps. According to Patrizio et al. (2022), facilitated by the accelerating development of ART, investors and several already existing physician groups striving for further national expansion have been racing towards the establishment of large international chains of fertility clinics. Two types of business models will be examined: (a) expansions and ongoing practice growth owned by doctors (type I model); (b) private investment firms entering the ART market through acquisition of existing ART practices and merging them into networks (type II model), in which physicians remain employed after their "payout" and become stockholders. One example of model I and II is the chain of reproductive clinics Valencian Institute of Infertility (IVI, Spain) – Reproductive Medicine Associates (RMA, USA). Other examples of Model II are Fresenius (Germany), Prelude (Spain) – Inception (USA) and Create Fertility (UK), which will be discussed later. And (c) the establishment of new independent ART clinics, sponsored entirely by investors who employ reproductive endocrinologists to operate them profitably under incentive programs (type III model). The new investors assert that they defer to physicians' judgements regarding clinical practice. However, they are revolutionizing a sector that has long been dominated by independent clinics (Robbins, 2017). The investment boom in the sector confirms that the fertility business continues to seduce private capital, the main protagonist. In the case of Spain, the appetite for the sector is motivated by several reasons: Spain leads the number of treatments in Europe which, together with the growing social demand and the existing liquidity in the private equity sector, are facilitating sales between pan-European and international funds (González, 2022).

Chains of fertility clinics: IVI (Spain) – RMA (USA)

In February 2017, the Valencian Institute of Infertility (IVI) in Spain merged with Reproductive Medicine Associates (RMA), founded by physicians in the United States, creating a global brand mostly on both sides of the Atlantic, IVI-RMA Global. IVI was founded in 1990 by Dr. Remohí and Dr. Pellicer, who remain shareholders and continue to run the business. In addition, they own subsidiaries in genetic testing, IVF lab consulting, research and development, and stem cell banking (IVI, 2023). IVI reported that they own 70% of the new company, while RMA owns 30%. The company includes 200 physicians and 300 research scientists across 70 clinics in 13 countries including Spain, the United Kingdom, Portugal, Turkey, Italy, Panama, Chile, Brazil, Argentina, and India (Patrizio et al., 2022). In 2019, IVI-RMA hired Morgan Stanley (investment banking, USA) to review strategic options for the company. The group aimed to get a US or Asian partner to help in expansion and take advantage of the growing demand for fertility treatment. Morgan Stanley handled the initial public offering (IPO) of another fertility company – Jinxin Fertility – on the Hong Kong Stock Exchange in June 2019.

IVI-RMA forecast €70 million in core profit EBITDA (earnings before interest, taxes, depreciation, and amortization), which is a widely used measure of core corporate profitability and was aiming for a valuation of 20 times that (Bayón & Martín Simón, 2019). Another notorious corporate operation in 2021 in the Spanish fertility market was the bid for the company Igenomix, a global leader in genetic tests for assisted reproduction clinics, valued at €1,000m. It was created in 2012 as a spin-off of IVI (Spain) and worked in parallel with two scenarios: its jump to the New York Stock Exchange and the Nasdaq advised by JP Morgan and Morgan Stanley (Bayón, 2021). Morgan Stanley reported solid results with net revenues of $13.1 billion (Morgan Stanley, 2022). In March 2022, the private equity manager KKR (USA) won the bid for IVI-RMA in an operation that values the company at approximately €3 billion (Web Capital Riesgo, 2022). Thus, IVI-RMA is the world's largest company exclusively devoted to human assisted reproduction technology (ART) with a presence in Spain and the United States, its main markets, as well as other countries. In 2021, IVI-RMA acquired "Create Fertility" in the United Kingdom, which had been founded in 2008 by Professor Geeta Nargund, a UK provider of reproductive treatments. The deal saw IVI-RMA take a majority stake in Create Fertility. KKR's goal was to merge IVI-RMA with its subsidiary GeneraLife, the third largest assisted reproduction company in Europe, to create a global fertility giant. The process was led by Morgan Stanley (USA) and Arcano (asset management, Spain), undertaken through private equity in the healthcare sector (Casado, 2021, 2022).

Chains of fertility clinics: GeneraLife (Spain), Fresenius (Germany), Create Fertility (UK)

In November 2021, KKR entered the fertility sector in Spain with the purchase of GeneraLife and Investindustrial in a process advised by Morgan Stanley. In order to build a sizable assisted reproduction group in southern Europe, Investindustrial started a build-up process before selling GeneraLife. This strategy involved gaining weight for the investee firm by the purchase of additional complimentary enterprises. In 2020, the chain of fertility clinics agreed to purchase Ginemed (Spain) for more than €50m. With this operation, GeneraLife became the third European group specializing in assisted reproduction. This key step in its growth strategy came after previously completing the acquisition of seven companies: Spain (Ginefiv and Ginemed), Czech Republic (FertiCare), Italy (Genera, Livet & Demetra), and Sweden (Linne) in just two years (Bravo, 2021). Elsewhere, Fresenius, a German company, one of the largest in-hospital and ambulatory service operators in Europe with properties in Germany, Spain, and Latin America, bought NMC Eugin Group (Spain), a company founded by a wealthy Indian billionaire residing in Dubai, who had been consolidating fertility clinics across Europe before entering the US market. By 2019, the Eugin Group was a European leader within the sector, with a team comprising over 1,000 specialists. In 2020, the Eugin Group was sold for €430m to Fresenius (EBIDTA 11.5x^2) (IMAP M&A Consultants AG, 2021). At the time of the sale, the Eugin Group's network comprised 31 ART clinics and

34 additional sites across 9 countries on 3 continents (Fresenius, 2020). Stephan Sturm, CEO of Fresenius said: "Eugin and Fresenius are an excellent fit. Eugin is highly profitable and holds excellent positions in attractive country markets". Dr. de Meo, CEO of Fresenius, added: "Eugin is an ideal addition to our portfolio as an integrated healthcare provider (…) thanks to our expertise and high success rates" (Fresenius, 2020).

Chains of fertility clinics: Prelude (Spain) – Inception (USA)

Top Silicon Valley companies like Google, Apple, and Facebook offer egg freezing as a benefit to employees, while some clinics host "egg socials" with wine and hors d'oeuvres to inform women of its advantages (Weller, 2017). According to Collins Ward, partner at the firm Lee Equity (USA), all that marketing, along with the aggressive expansion push, has "added significant costs". Due to the possibility of an exponential increase gain, Lee Equity has been willing to invest in them. Data demonstrating the escalating average age of first-time mothers in the United States initially drew the attention of the financial officers at Lee Equity to the field of fertility. The legalization of same-sex marriage has also attracted their interest, since it might increase the number of couples looking for reproductive services. In the United States, one cycle of IVF costs an average of $12,000, but the price can rise to $22,000 with additional treatments. However, as they began investigating the field, they found the potential market was larger still: "Probably the biggest surprise to us as we started to work on our investment thesis in this industry was just how low awareness is of fertility services, not only IVF, but also egg freezing, as well as donor eggs", stated Ward (Robbins, 2017). Thus, Lee Equity backed the serial entrepreneur Martin Varsavsky (Spain), who created his fortune through telephone companies in Spain, with $200m when he launched into the fertility business in the United States with the company "Prelude", setting up assisted reproduction clinics that joined the company "Inception" (USA), with clinics across 23 states. Prelude is already the first chain of fertility clinics in the United States that offers comprehensive services (from genetic tests to all kinds of reproductive treatments). Varsavsky's other company, "Overture Life", is perfecting a robot that produces viable embryos. He has also invested in companies like the Google-backed "23andMe", which does genetic testing, with a $13.1m investment (Investors 23andme, 2022). Collins Ward, the partner at Lee Equity who led the investment in Prelude, built this company in part to help its newly acquired clinics revamp their marketing strategy. Dr. Mehmet Oz, host of "The Dr. Oz Show" in the United States, sits on Prelude's board of directors (Terry, 2016). Dr. Oz describes himself as a Republican, and opposes abortion and the Affordable Care Act, thus creating a conflict of interest for Dr. Oz: abortion laws might effectively also ban in vitro fertilization. Dr. Oz was appointed by former president Donald Trump to his council on sport, fitness, and nutrition in 2020. Both promoted the use of hydroxychloroquine, an antimalarial drug, as a cure for COVID-19 (Caulfield, 2020). According to his financial disclosure, Dr. Oz and his wife hold between $1.5m and $6m of shares in Prelude (Kilgore, 2022).

Fertility events: marketing, business, and client acquisition

In 2019, "The Economist" published an article entitled, "The fertility business is booming" (The Economist, 2019). A year earlier, in October 2018, I described in my field diary my visit to an event in London (UK) called "Pathways to Parenthood", held in partnership with the private London Women's Clinic, which consists of nine clinics, and whose main clinic is located on Harley Street, a global hub for private healthcare. The event was also organized by Bindmans LLP solicitors, which focused on donor and surrogacy families. They joined forces with the London Women's Clinic to host this evening seminar with the aim: "to bring clarity to the medical and legal processes involved in creating a modern family, with additional information from the London Egg Bank, London Sperm Bank and support organisations". The event promised that the evening would provide us with all we needed to know as we approached parenthood, principally motherhood since the majority were women, approximately 85 out of 90 people. This event was sponsored by the charity "Fertility Network", which offers support to more than 3.5 million people facing fertility issues in the United Kingdom. This charity is backed by a network of professionals from across the fertility industry: fertility clinics and corporate organizations. It receives funding from The National Lottery Community Fund for England and Wales, which is a non-departmental public body responsible for distributing funds raised by the National Lottery for "good causes" (National Lottery Funding, 2022), and from the Scottish government, sharing good practice with Health Boards in Scotland. They also receive funding from the Health & Social Care Board in Northern Ireland (Fertility Network, 2022). This event was therefore financed with public money and organized by a private group of fertility clinics and a law firm. The seminar was held in a hall in central London, and huge posters with smiling babies welcomed us. Advertising scholars Tushnet and Goldman (2014) state that an effect of images of babies is that the images might suggest the outcome of treatment: a successful pregnancy. They stress that advertising that uses visual elements and lets consumers make their own inferences are more persuasive to consumers than those that make explicit assertions or use verbal metaphors.

Patients are more likely to act on information if they see children and establish a relationship between the treatment and pregnancy on their own. Images of successful pregnancies may therefore be even more convincing than the frequently made statements about the success rates of clinics. These smiling babies were accompanied by the logo of the clinic and the law firm, visual identifiers that promote their brands by repeatedly associating meaning with them. The London Women's Clinic is one of the leading fertility clinics in Britain that treats self-funded and National Health Service (NHS) patients and is licensed by the Human Fertilisation and Embryology Authority (HFEA), the UK Fertility Regulator. Hawkins argues that:

> Another category of advertising that clinics [...] rely on is advertising based on third-party assessments of the clinics. [...] Third-party assessments in the

> first three classifications are significant from a practical standpoint because patients may lack the ability or knowledge to assess what clinic is best for them.
>
> (2013, p. 1159)

Studies reveal that customers give board certification a lot of consideration when choosing a doctor. Board certification, membership in professional organizations, and endorsements can also serve as trustmarks (Sage, 1999). On the tables at the event there were snacks and goody bags: bags with the logo of the clinic that contained a book edited by the clinic explaining the benefits of its assisted reproduction treatments, highlighting its success rates. The room was full of comfortable chairs for potential clients: the fertility business offered hope to people struggling to conceive and extended that promise to solo women, to same-sex couples, and increasingly to young women who want to postpone childbearing by freezing their eggs. In addition to using these types of advertising, clinics market themselves using information about the medical services they offer: (1) excellent technology; (2) personal, caring treatment; and (3) high-quality doctors (Hawkins, 2013). One of the speakers from the clinic asserted that: "the clinic offers lots of support before, during and after treatment, an amazing, brilliant team of doctors that are there seven days a week". Women's testimonies, which I analyze later, contrast with this statement. Thus, this publicly funded event confirmed that the ART business aroused the interest not only of clinics (private and public) but also of law firms and as many industries (i.e., pharmaceutical companies) and organizations (i.e., charities) as necessary to offer a pack to the clientele for which they need to pay separately.

According to Krawiec (2009) in the case of the United States: "Doubtless, a desire to help infertile couples is a motivating factor for many doctors, reproductive center directors, counselors, and others involved in the fertility industry. But profits are undeniably a – if not the – motivating factor in the reproductive industry". And the same applies in the case of the United Kingdom (Howard, 2018) and Spain (Immedico, 2023). The fertility clinic itself is frequently a professionally managed, for-profit, private organization, even though many fertility clinics are associated with non-profit hospitals or university institutions. Those fertility clinics that are not affiliated with academic institutions are even more overtly profit-driven and, like suppliers in any competitive market, they use extensive marketing strategies to draw in clients: "hiring high-priced marketing consultants; advertising on billboards, the radio, newspapers, and magazines; and assiduously courting physician referrals by 'wining and dining' doctors and hosting dinners and parties at medical meetings" (Krawiec, 2009, p. 13). As a result, the fertility industry is a market where customers make decisions. Although it may be challenging to distinguish between patients and consumers in the context of people seeking fertility treatments because they function as both, the consumer aspect of interactions between clinics and patients is crucial because patients have the freedom to choose their own healthcare provider. In a medicalized, consumer-based paradigm, clinics are focused on treating patients/customers. The features that clinics choose to advertise might reveal the factors they think patients use to decide which clinic to select for reproductive treatment (Cahn, 2012).

Consumer law, national commissions, personal gain, and ethical standards

The Competition and Markets Authority (CMA) review regarding the fertility clinics' compliance with consumer law in the United Kingdom found a mixed picture: patients are not always getting the information they need to make informed decisions. In 2020, the CMA raised concerns about some practices by fertility clinics, such as providing unclear price information and advertising misleading success rates. It also identified a general lack of awareness that consumer law applies in the sector. The report stated that compliance issues were found with the majority of clinics reviewed (CMA, 2022). The provision of accurate, clear, and transparent information upfront is critical for patients, particularly regarding prices and success rates. The way in which patients fund their treatment varies widely, from using their savings, gifts from parents, loans from siblings, personal loans, credit cards, inheritance, or redundancy pay-outs to re-mortgaging their house, or often a combination of these. Most patients buying fertility treatment for the first time carry out a shortlisting process, primarily online using clinic websites, and mainly factoring in clinics' location, prices, and success rates. Significant differences exist between what clinics include in their package for a single cycle of IVF, making it very difficult for patients to compare prices when shortlisting clinics. As part of its next steps, the CMA planned to hold roundtable discussions with clinics and the sector, including the Human Fertilisation and Embryology Authority (HFEA), to explore the feasibility of developing a standard approach for what is included in the headline package price, so patients can meaningfully compare clinics. Rachel Cutting, Director of Compliance at the HFEA, said: "Both regulators (HFEA and CMA) have recognised that making decisions about fertility treatment, where most patients are paying for it themselves, can be expensive and difficult, as well as emotionally and physically draining" (HFEA, 2022a). However, the website of the HFEA asserts that they provide:

> Impartial, accurate information about clinics and fertility treatments from the UK government fertility regulator. Our board – 'the Authority' – is made up of appointed members, who are people we've chosen for their expertise and knowledge to bring an objective viewpoint to decision making.
>
> (HFEA, 2022b)

Yet one of the board members is Professor Child, who is the medical and founding director of TFP Oxford Fertility, a group of 20 private clinics in 6 European countries (TFP, 2022). Another board member is Professor Nargund, the medical director of Create Fertility, with 16 private clinics across the United Kingdom and Denmark (Create Fertility, 2022). Create Fertility, as I mentioned earlier, was bought in 2021 by IVI (Spain)-RMA (USA) with the help of KKR (private equity, USA). Create Fertility collaborates with private sperm banks such as: Create Fertility (UK), Cryos

International (Denmark), and the European Sperm Bank (Denmark). Clients who require egg donation are suggested to go to Spain. How can the HFEA claim to be an "independent, objective and impartial authority" when several of its members belong to corporate holdings of private fertility clinics that serve their own and their shareholders' economic interests?

Patients deserve to be represented nationally by an organization that fully reflects high ethical standards that are not biased by personal financial gain over patients' reproductive health needs (Brody, 2010). "The public must feel confident that national health organizations will offer only those proposals that will improve the health of the public" (Kass, 2001, p. 209). Private actors may not be in a position to provide "public goods" and they may operate under biased information. In the case of Spain, the National Commission for Assisted Human Reproduction (CNRHA, 2022), which belongs to the Spanish Ministry of Health, some of the members are also directors of private reproductive clinics, such as Dr. Llácer, who is the medical director of Ginefiv GeneraLife Clinics (described earlier) with 16 private clinics in Spain and a total of 53 private clinics in Europe. KKR acquired GeneraLife for €400 million in November 2021. KKR co-chairman and co-CEO George Roberts states that: "As investors with an industrialist vision we aim to generate attractive investment returns" (KKR, 2022). Dr. Llácer is also vice-president of the Spanish Fertility Society and was a Member of the Committee of National Representatives of the European Society of Human Reproduction and Embryology. Another vocal member of the CNRHA is Dr. Urries, Director of the Assisted Reproduction Unit of the private Hospital Quirón Salud Zaragoza, and president of the Association for the Study of Reproductive Biology (CNRHA, 2022). How is it possible that several members of this national commission are directors of private clinics whose objective is to seek profit? What are the ethical implications? What are their biases when deciding the regulation of assisted reproduction in Spain? As Sherrie A. Kossoudji (2005, p. 26) wrote almost two decades ago: "while we argue ethics, the markets go on, fed by technology, need, altruism and greed".

Women's perspectives

Most of the participants in this study had to resort to private healthcare for the following reasons: (a) the long waiting lists in public hospitals; (b) solo women were placed behind heterosexual couples on the waiting list; (c) some gynecologists, in public and private clinics, denied them treatment since they only considered heterosexual couples; and (d) they were "advanced in age", 35 years or older, and this would affect the success rates of the clinic, that is, these women had fewer chances of getting pregnant. None of the women interviewed was offered psychological support in the private or public clinics that treated self-funded patients, regardless of the age at which they conceived or the decade in which they were treated. That is, neither the oldest participant over 65 years of age, British, who gave birth in 1995, nor the Spanish participant to whom an embryo had just been transferred in 2021. Thus, for more than two decades these women were not offered any psychological support in Spain or the United Kingdom, despite the fact that most of them had gone through multiple failed attempts to become pregnant, miscarriages, embryonic reduction, some suffered from depression and anxiety before treatment, some were alone without family or friends' support, and some had to confront their families' opposition to their reproductive treatment. Most studies have conducted research on infertile heterosexual couples and conclude that the cost and psychological burden of treatment were the main reasons cited for discontinuation before achieving a birth. Discontinuation rates were as high as 13%–60% between consecutive cycles (de la Rochebrochard et al., 2008; Gameiro et al., 2013; McDowell & Murray, 2011; Miller et al., 2021; Schröder et al., 2004; Troude et al., 2014). Pasch et al. (2016), who conducted a prospective longitudinal cohort study in the United States in five fertility clinics with a total of 352 women and 274 men seeking treatment for infertility, concluded that psychological distress is common during fertility treatment. However, most patients do not receive counselling and are not referred to mental health services (MHS); moreover, referral is not targeted at those at high risk of serious psychological distress.

Patients' depression and anxiety that clinics ignore

Mila, 38 years old, French, who arrived in London 20 years ago, and has a three-month-old son, works in human resources and is a self-declared Roman Catholic. At the age of 32 she decided she wanted to pursue motherhood on her own and paid privately for her treatment because there was a long waiting list at the NHS hospital:

> I had less than 0.5% chance to conceive with my own eggs. I had a past of health issues and a cyst. The first attempt was with my own eggs, I had three transfers of embryos and became pregnant twice but did not result in a baby. I had two miscarriages. Then I had a double donation from an egg donor from the UK and a sperm donor from abroad and became pregnant with my son. It took me literally six years to get pregnant. It hurts more than anything, psychologically. I had suffered from depression, I've been now off medication for three years. But I was on medication, and being treated by a therapist privately. First I was scared my depression would hinder my pregnancy. Then, I literally ticked all the boxes for severe post-natal depression. For a long time, I was preparing myself economically, mentally, emotionally, spiritually for the reproductive treatment.

Mila revealed that she privately paid for a therapist who helped her overcome her depression also through the six-year process of getting pregnant, and overcoming failed pregnancy attempts and miscarriages. At no time did the clinic offer psychological support or suggest that she have it, despite the fact that she had informed the clinic of her history of depression. Another participant is Martine, a 53-year-old physiotherapist from Belgium, Roman Catholic, who has lived in London for the past 25 years. Her son is 10 years old and was conceived with anonymous donor sperm and her eggs at a private clinic, due to a long waiting list at the NHS hospital. Initially her parents and sister disapproved of her reproductive treatment due to religious reasons. Her mother thought it was wrong for her to choose this type of family "without a father for the child". Her sister said to her: "You are a bad influence on my children", and thinks of her as selfish. Once the baby was born her parents were thrilled about their grandson. Her sister did not change her mind. She had to undergo seven IVF attempts over a five-year period. After the sixth attempt with the same hospital, they told her to go somewhere else. She went to another hospital owned by the Hospital Corporation of America (HCA), the largest private operator of healthcare facilities in the world, and one of the leading private healthcare providers in the United Kingdom. On her seventh attempt she became pregnant with her son. They transferred three embryos. Only one survived:

> I've got a big tendency of being depressed and anxious, but I kind of love life. My self-esteem will be very low and I'll be very anxious and thinking, 'I'm so crap at everything.' I had a lot of therapy to help me with that and I still have periods where I am depressed. There was a time when I was pregnant when I would think, 'Have I done the right thing? How am I going to cope?' I was really quite worried at times. I didn't really share that much, because I guess unconsciously, I felt, 'I can't really tell people it's hard work, because I chose to be a solo mum'.

This is another case in which the patient underwent psychotherapy for her depression and anxiety. Both hospitals knew her medical history, but neither offered psychological support, despite six attempts to get pregnant that did not result in a birth. They did not care how she managed her failed treatments and her history of depression and anxiety. According to Sagili and Divers (2011): "Modern treatment of miscarriage should provide a rapid diagnosis, adequate counselling and access to appropriate information. It requires a dedicated multidisciplinary team ideally consisting of doctors, nurses and support staff". Pasch et al. (2012) argue that attention needs to be paid to helping patients prepare for and cope with treatment and treatment failure. The longitudinal studies that have examined psychological distress before and after reproductive treatment suggest that depression and anxiety increase after reproductive treatment failure, with about 10–25% of women at risk for clinically relevant distress after unsuccessful treatment. In a Dutch study, Verhaak et al. (2005) focused on 202 women who pursued pregnancy with their male partner and who initiated their first IVF cycle at any time during the 18-month study period (sperm donor, egg donor, and surrogacy cycles were excluded). Women whose IVF treatment was unsuccessful experienced an increase in depression and anxiety relative to their pre-IVF psychological status that persisted over the subsequent six months since their last attempt. Furthermore, 20% of the patients experienced anxiety and depression in the clinically relevant range. In contrast, women who became pregnant following IVF experienced a decrease in depression and anxiety over the same time period. Anxiety and depression reverted to pre-IVF levels over the subsequent three to five years in women who still did not have a baby, whereas women who did have a baby experienced improvements compared with pre-IVF levels. These findings suggest that psychological distress before and after reproductive treatment is a significant issue. Moreover, the profile of the sample for the present ethnographic study differs from Verhaak's target group as these women pursue motherhood on their own without the help of a partner and all of them needed at least a sperm donor to become pregnant. Furthermore, in the case of Mila and Martine they had to deal with their depression and anxiety at the same time as trying to get pregnant. Martine also had to deal with her family's hostility to her treatment and, as a result, her loneliness throughout this process.

Clinics as minefields: manipulation, profits, and success rates

Emerald is 65 years old, a Jewish white South African and a British citizen, who works as head of Midwifery at a public hospital in the United Kingdom, and gave birth 23 years ago:

> I lived in a borough that does not support a single woman having children. I was over 35, I had polycystic ovaries and I got no support. I could not access the NHS. I was single and clinics weren't interested. So, I had to pay for everything: I nearly bankrupted myself. I had to pay for all my own drugs and for all my own appointments. I got pregnant on my fifth attempt.

She used her own eggs and wanted a Jewish sperm donor. In her fertility clinic she saw two counsellors, the first one said it was not ethical to choose a sperm donor based on his religion. Then she changed counsellor in the same clinic, who said: "ethically it is not ideal but if that is your choice". Emerald argues that:

> Clinics will do anything to get you pregnant. I changed sperm donors halfway through because they wondered if that was part of the problem of my not getting pregnant. I then went home to South Africa and my nanny that was known as a sangoma,[1] which is like a witch doctor, and her specialty was infertility, gave me something to drink and I got pregnant on the next cycle. Psychological? Who knows … She said I had too many drugs in my system. The clinics make you menopausal in order to start a natural cycle. And I hyper-stimulated every cycle, I was making a lot of eggs. I hadn't told people, so nobody knew why I was so fat or why so unwell. I was going to the clinic, having my eggs removed and going straight to work. When you're desperate, as a lot of women will tell you, you'll do anything. I got pregnant on the fifth go having had a very big argument with the clinic, because I said I wanted to stop. You get very caught up in it. It becomes an emotional rollercoaster. For the clinics it's a financial investment. If they can get a 40-year-old pregnant, their stats go up. It's all about stats and money in those places. Things happened in that clinic that I think, if the HFEA knew, that clinic would have gotten into a lot of trouble. When I was there for the fifth attempt and I said: "this is the last time" the nurse told me: "Wait a minute" and she came back with a photograph of a mixed-race family: A mother,

> a father and three kids, and she said: "They've got spare embryos to give you if you want them". And I went: "Why?" and she said: "Because they've been in the freezer for five years and either they get chucked out or they go for research and they don't want them to go to research". And I replied: "What makes you think I want those embryos?", and she said: "You were desperate for a child", so I said: "Yes, but there's ethical and emotional issues". The nurse got quite cross. They would do things like insert the embryos and say: "We've got lucky fingers, we'll get you pregnant this time". I just hated that. Firstly, you're very emotional. Secondly, you're hormonal up to your eyeballs because I was so full of drugs. I'm allergic to estrogen and so it was really hard doing all of this. It was also very scary because I was doing it on my own.

As Emerald portrays, private enterprises with increasingly aggressive sales techniques are fueling growth in this for-profit medical field. However, market values might not be a good foundation for building families. Private clinics are expected to respond to investors seeking returns on their investments. Profits, and not patients, emerge as the principal priority, often to the detriment of cycle outcomes and patient satisfaction. Emerald states that the ethos of treating fertility medicine as a cash cow led her clinic to try to manipulate her, presenting her with two choices: an embryo she did not want, and another attempt at IVF with the "lucky fingers" of her nurse, whom she did not trust any more. These two options were to further pressurize Emerald into taking action then or else suffer the consequences: not having a baby. This is a deceitful technique of manipulation that is often used in high-stakes sales environments to get customers to take advantage of a limited-time-only deal (Bault & Rusconi, 2020). It is about creating tension that demands release, which Emerald would be granted if she agreed to her nurse's demands. "There's a fine line that must be walked to steer clear of preying on someone's emotions", says Dr. Ravi Gada, who co-owns Dallas Fort Worth Fertility Associates, which has turned away multiple overtures from private equity firms (Robbins, 2017).

It was in a similar scenario that, Lia, who is 43, a university lecturer from an Argentine family exiled in Madrid, was treated in a private clinic with her own egg and sperm from an anonymous donor. Her son was born 3 years ago. Lia emphasizes that the clinics are businesses: "the more tests and services you get, the more you pay and the more profit they make". For this reason, she investigated different clinics to avoid being deceived by them selling her a pack of tests and services she did not need. Having done her research she went to the clinic of her choice:

> I visited different private clinics, due to my age I could not access the NHS. I took tests to know what situation I and my eggs were in. I had many doubts because the clinics are a business and they generated a lot of insecurity in me … they are there to get money and the more the better. For that reason I consulted four clinics and independent gynecologists, so that the clinic I finally chose wouldn't try to sell me a pack I did not need.

According to Goodwin et al. (2019), there are three things needed for a market to function effectively: (a) you need to have choice (competition); (b) transparency, that is, you know what you are getting and what the benefit of the bargain is; and (c) that there is no conflict of interest. In the ART business, clinics fail on the last two grounds. Lia refers to corporate greed: reproductive clinics opportunistically may try to take advantage of a situation to strictly serve their best interests (i.e., profit) in a way that is detrimental to the patient (Bies & Tripp, 2009; Crossley, 2009). Such uncaring treatment angers Lia to the extent that she becomes ethically outraged. She employed the tactic of talking with independent doctors before selecting a clinic in an effort to stop the practices of greedy clinics. Patients expect clinics to have ethical obligations to consider patients' well-being in the field of (reproductive) medicine. When patients perceive an intentional violation of these obligations, they may infer that the clinic acts with the goal of profiting financially and not in the best interests of the patient.

Failed attempts, miscarriages, and grief: no psychological support

Sophie who is 54 years old, from London, and works as a criminal lawyer, has a ten-year-old boy. She was treated privately at an NHS Hospital in London:

> At the time the hospital was trying to get a licence from HFEA to import sperm from Denmark. Age was a big thing and also the fact that I was going to be a single parent. They said: "We can put you on our waiting list but you'll come behind all the couples". It was only three years after the changes in law (2005) and there was no donor sperm in London. I'd phoned around all the private clinics and they all said, " 'We've got no sperm donors". I had 3 times IUI and I had one miscarriage when I was 9 weeks pregnant. Then I went to Copenhagen and tried IUI which was not successful. I also tried one IVF there, they transferred two embryos, one didn't succeed but the other one is my son.

Agenor and Bhattacharya (2015) argue that women undergoing assisted reproductive treatment are at a greater risk of having a miscarriage, especially at an advanced age, compared with women conceiving naturally. Nearly 30% of embryos are lost upon implantation, making human reproduction an inefficient process. At post-implantation, but before the first missed menstruation, 30% of biochemical pregnancies are lost. After the first missed menstruation, 10% of embryos are lost and are termed clinical miscarriage (Bottomley & Bourne, 2009). Furthermore, miscarriage is common after undergoing fertility treatments. If pregnancy is defined as commencing at the time of implantation, pregnancy wastage can occur at any time after the blastocyst implants in the uterus. According to Agenor and Bhattacharya (2015) over the age of 40 years, only 50% of women are still capable of conceiving and the risk of miscarriage is five times greater than women aged between 31 and 35 years. Hu et al. (2018) state that more than one embryo transfer is a protective factor against fetal loss in ART pregnancies after accounting for maternal age and the transfer of two embryos is associated with a significant decreased risk of early loss.

Another case is that of Louise, from London, who is 50 years old and gave birth to her son two years ago. She is the director of a research company, and paid over £30,000 for IVF over a four-year period. Louise also points to the shortage of donors due to the non-anonymity law (2005) in the United Kingdom. She bought sperm online from Xytex, a Sperm Bank in Atlanta (USA). She comments:

> Which clinic? [...] It's quite a minefield to navigate. After four goes, actually I got pregnant, first time there was nothing. Second time, I had a chemical pregnancy for a few days, it looks like you might be pregnant, but you're not, and then the third time I got pregnant, but I had a miscarriage after seven weeks, and then my sister donated me her eggs, so the fourth time was all good.

Neither Sophie nor Louise were offered psychological support, despite the miscarriages, the failed attempts, and the number of years of reproductive treatment that caused multiple feelings of grief. First, in Louise's case, she was unable to become pregnant with her own eggs, which led her to suffer from genetic grief. This is the emotional reaction of loss when the reception of donor eggs or embryos is considered the only possibility of becoming a biological mother. Second, both of them got pregnant but it did not result in a birth: they suffered from gestational grief – namely grief experienced by women who undergo treatment without being able to become pregnant. And third, because in the case of Louise, she had a miscarriage in the seventh week of gestation and suffered from gestational loss. During the four years that this process lasted, the clinics in London and Copenhagen only prescribed medication and applied ART treatments. The clinics ignored the psychological pain that Sophie and Louise suffered. Psychological support before, during, and after ART is crucial for the management of psychosocial aspects that characterize the grief process of women trying to become pregnant, women who cannot use their own eggs and suffer miscarriages (de Castro et al., 2021; Lukse & Vacc, 1999; Reardon, 2018). The findings of Boivin et al. (2011) and Matthiesen et al. (2011) do suggest an urgent need to reduce the stress of ART and to help patients cope with treatment and treatment failure. As argued by Boivin and colleagues, these efforts must be targeted and address multiple domains, including patient factors as well as clinic and treatment factors (Boivin et al., 2012). Clinic and treatment factors are important so that the burden of stress reduction is not placed solely on the patient, but instead shared by the physicians, nurses, laboratory personnel, billing staff, and pharmaceutical companies. For example, research has suggested that perhaps some treatment protocols might be associated with lower distress while maintaining pregnancy rates (de Klerk et al., 2006), and that interventions can be targeted at all patients at specific points along the treatment process by specific staff (i.e., phones calls from nurses during the waiting period) (Lancastle & Boivin, 2008). The development of intervention strategies to reduce stress and improve coping is important to attain the goal of reducing emotional suffering (Domar et al., 2010; Zareba et al., 2020).

Import of gametes: every woman to herself

In the case of Nina, 39, a Spanish resident in London who works for an NGO, she had an embryo transferred in 2020. She has endometriosis, suffered a miscarriage with an ex-partner, and later had a molar[2] pregnancy. When she decided to become a mother on her own, she went to a private clinic in London. At her initial appointment, the embryologist treated her condescendingly because she did not have a partner. When she went to pay for her consultation, they told her that she could have a test at that moment to find out what her ovarian reserve was, which cost £400. Nina complains:

> As if anyone had £400 to spend at once! As if it were a pint of beer! The deal seemed absolutely commercial to me, they were trying to get the money out of you however they could. Despite the fact that this clinic was one of the best according to its success rates on the HFEA website. So I went to a second clinic that was Spanish (IVI) in London. There was a waiting list for sperm donors in the UK and I didn't want to wait, nor did I want sperm from a Danish bank. I didn't want to have a blond child with blue eyes, since I am a brunette with brown eyes. I decided on the Cryobank bank, in California, the clinic suggested it to me. The more information I wanted to know about the donors, the more I had to pay to Cryobank: photos from when they were little, when they were older, an essay written by them, an audio recording ... I bought and imported the sperm that arrived at Heathrow airport (London). It got lost at the airport and later found. The clinic did not take responsibility for the importation.

Commoditization that results from industrialization compels doctors to spend less time with patients, and promotes expensive treatments even when more affordable alternatives are also acceptable. According to Connolly, Hoorens, Chambers (2010, p. 603):

> The direct costs of ART treatment vary substantially between countries (and regions). The direct costs generally reflect the costliness of the underlying healthcare system. If unsubsidized, direct costs represent a significant economic burden to patients. The level of affordability of ART treatment is an important driver of utilization and treatment choices.

In addition, a study by Cambridge University that looked at 67 countries across the world stated that family physicians' consultations in Britain are among the shortest in Europe. It concludes that short consultations "adversely affect patient care" (Irving et al., 2017).

Nina was surprised that the embryologist treated her condescendingly and that she suggested paying £400 for a test, the same test that cost €38 in a private clinic in Spain (Quirón Salud, 2022). It should also be noted that neither Cryobank nor the IVI clinic in London ensured that the sperm Nina had purchased on the clinic's advice reached the clinic safely. This is in spite of the huge profits that both companies make: Cryobank, is a leading provider of gametes for fertility treatments and was acquired for approximately $1.6 billion by Cooper Companies from GeneraLife (Cooper Companics, 2021). IVI-RMA is worth up to €2 billion (Burgos, 2022). Neither company took responsibility for the importation of sperm that Nina bought at the risk of losing it at Heathrow airport.

Another case is that of Marta, 33, from Madrid, who works in human resources and has a ten-month-old baby. Marta could not access an NHS hospital because of the legislation at the time excluding solo women and lesbians from assisted reproduction treatments, legislation which was passed by the conservative party (Partido Popular) that governed in Madrid. In a private clinic she underwent six IUI inseminations with her eggs and sperm imported from Copenhagen. She had four miscarriages:

> I found out through a sperm bank in Copenhagen that they exported to some clinics in Madrid, so I went to one of those clinics and told them I wanted a non-anonymous sperm donor. The clinic told me to import the sperm from the bank in Denmark which arrived in Barajas airport and I collected it and took it to the clinic.

The clinic in Madrid ignored Marta's suffering caused by her four miscarriages throughout the treatment performed at that clinic. They did not prepare her for treatment failure, or help her to cope with it. Verhaak et al. (2007) argue that the availability of psychological counselling services was vitally important at times of distress. The authors state that ongoing counselling should be part of having reproductive treatment and that the clinic should contact patients between treatments because in their sample only a small proportion of the women availed themselves of the counselling services beyond the initial counselling session. On the contrary, it was already known that the most distressed patients fail to initiate contact with counsellors (Boivin et al., 1999). There should therefore be a reassessment of individuals' feelings and degree of psychological distress after each reproductive treatment cycle (Guerra et al., 1998). Furthermore, neither the sperm bank in Copenhagen nor the clinic in Madrid took responsibility for the import–export process, leaving it up to chance that the gametes reached the clinic safely, causing even more stress and concern to Marta.

Some clinics' negligence and lack of ethics

Ainhoa, a 45-year-old Spanish web developer from Madrid, had her baby at the age of 42 with a double donation. One of her ovaries had been removed at the age of 19. When she was 42 she had her eggs retrieved for IVF at a clinic in Madrid through private insurance, but they were only able to retrieve one egg and she did not get pregnant. The second time, they retrieved three eggs and two embryos were transferred. However, she lost one embryo very soon after implantation and then she had a miscarriage at nine weeks. In a check-up they saw that the baby's heart was not beating. She was informed that she could have an abortion by taking abortion pills. She asserts that it was traumatic. She was sent home when she was in a lot of pain. She later returned to the clinic to request an aspiration curettage because of the intense pain she felt, but they told her that she had already taken the pills and that they could not do it:

> Alone, at home, I suffered an abortion caused by the pills, which was horrible, psychologically and physically traumatic. I was left with a lot of pain every time I had my period. At another hospital they diagnosed me with a nodule and they had to cut my rectum. A year later I adopted an embryo at another clinic, I tried twice but it didn't work. I had two miscarriages. My last attempt was at another clinic with a double donation of frozen gametes, a cheaper option, from a Spanish egg donor and a Danish sperm donor. Fortunately I got pregnant.

None of the three clinics offered her psychological support. Ainhoa only had one ovary left and she was 42 years old when she had her eggs retrieved. Studies suggest that women whose eggs are retrieved before the age of 35 have a better chance of a successful pregnancy. A woman's fertility declines with age. That decline accelerates in her late thirties due to a sharp decrease in both the quantity and quality of available eggs. As women age, their risk of miscarriages, chromosomal abnormalities, and trouble conceiving increases. To ensure healthy and viable eggs, some fertility experts suggest limiting elective egg retrieval to women aged 38 years and under (University of Pittsburgh Medical Center, 2021). Thus, considering Ainhoa's age and medical history, was it ethical to advise her to have an egg retrieval procedure? The scenario may change when there are more public fertility clinics and more insurance companies that cover fertility services. Such initiatives might provide women with access to evidence-based treatments without incurring astronomical costs and would be less likely to be motivated by the need to return profits to private equity firms or pay dividends to shareholders.

Gala, a Spanish social worker who lives in a small city in Spain, had frozen her eggs at the age of 39 on the advice of the specialist at a private clinic. She had undergone hormonal treatment and the egg retrieval produced five eggs of which only two turned out to be of good quality. At 44, she decided she wanted to be a mother and they fertilized the two frozen eggs with anonymous donor sperm, transferred them to her and a few weeks later they observed she had lost the embryos:

> I felt completely devastated, deeply sad. I thought that since I had frozen my eggs at 39 I had a good chance that they would result in a pregnancy. It was very painful, not only had I lost both embryos, but I would not be able to get pregnant with my eggs in the future. I had assumed that I would be a mother with my own eggs and now I had to manage my grief. Soon after I decided to become a mother with a double donation in another clinic. The specialist who had treated

> me was always travelling to international conferences and we were in contact by e-mail, I felt very helpless. So I went to another clinic and the gynecologist transferred me two embryos even though I only wanted one, but she said that I had a better chance of one surviving if they transferred me two. In a check-up they told me that I was pregnant with two and I felt a lot of joy and a lot of panic at the same time. I could only have one due to my personal circumstances. Then the gynecologist referred me to another clinic in another city because they did not do embryo reductions for religious reasons! Nobody at that clinic had informed me about this before starting my treatment! I felt devastated: I had frozen my eggs, I had lost the possibility of being a mother with my eggs, two embryos had been transferred to me by double donation and now I risked losing both in the embryo reduction procedure. Words cannot describe the heartbreak, fear and loneliness of this whole process. At no point did either of the three clinics offered me psychological support. I paid for three sessions with a psychologist specializing in assisted reproduction who helped me manage my genetic grief. Fortunately, after this hard and painful journey, I had my daughter.

In the first clinic she only saw the gynecologist once, after which they kept in touch by e-mail. She experienced the way she was treated as "barely humane" and felt helpless when she was unable to get pregnant with the eggs she had frozen. Gala went to another clinic that did not inform her that they would not perform an embryo reduction in the event that she became pregnant with two, despite the fact that Gala had told them from the beginning that she could only have one baby. Therefore, the clinic hid information from her so that she would not choose another clinic where they practiced assisted reproduction and embryo reduction. Gala had to go to a third clinic in another city where they performed an embryo reduction, and where she had to sign a document informing her that she could lose both embryos. None of the three clinics offered her psychological support; she had to manage her genetic grief by paying a psychologist out of her own pocket. Moreover, the second and third clinic disregarded the fear and pain Gala felt when she learned that she could end up not having a baby.

Reflections

This chapter has presented the economic context of assisted reproduction, an industry that is worth billions and from which chains of assisted reproduction clinics are backed by large private investment companies that expect profits. These clinics are mostly led by doctors who also may have profits from other related industries and who become physician-entrepreneurs whose scientific, medical, and business interests overlap. Furthermore, the purpose of marketing is to generate revenue, and deceptive marketing uses misleading information to capture the attention of the consumer through the use of false information. In the case of ART clinics, they inflate the "success rates" of treatments and fail to offer transparent information so that the patient can have a clear idea of the total price of each treatment from the beginning. This entails trying to convince patients to enter into a business transaction that will often be advantageous for clinics rather than the patient. At no time these patients were informed of the possible consequences of assisted reproduction treatment: failed attempts, miscarriages, embryo reduction, side effects of hormones, or the years of attempts that may be needed to get pregnant. Moreover, in this process patients may feel different types of grief, sometimes cumulative, for which neither public nor private clinics provide psychological support. This conflict of interest – medical and business – is reflected in the clinics and in the experiences of these women who complain that the clinics are a business, that they do not know if they sell them treatments or tests because they need them or to increase the clinics' profit margins to keep investors satisfied. Furthermore, the national commissions that regulate assisted reproduction in both countries have appointed members who lead chains of private clinics. These members' economic interests generate an ethical conflict, yet they are part of the national commissions linked to respective ministries of public health whose objective should be to look after the common good. In addition, NHS hospitals that treat self-funded patients are financed mainly from general taxation supplemented by national insurance contributions. Even private hospitals like the Quirón network of hospitals in Spain mediated by multi-insurance groups like ASISA or ADESLAS obtain state subsidies to potentially treat 17% of the population, almost 3 million workers, that are publicly employed (Eurostat, 2018). NHS hospitals and private clinics also profit from medical research and medical education paid for by taxpayers' money. Thus, mixing business with medicine may lead to abuses that violate patients' trust, as has been shown in this chapter. A patient may be in a vulnerable position, necessarily trusting that the doctor's decisions about her medical care will be guided solely by the patient's best interests. In a system of for-profit assisted reproductive medicine, doctors may become accountable to shareholders whose primary aim is to make a profit. Such hospitals and clinics may encourage doctors to promote profit-producing medicines, tests, and treatments. Thus, medical treatments and counselling that lack profit potential, however effective, are discouraged. This is the case of the psychological care that patients need in the process of getting pregnant and having a baby through assisted reproduction. Despite the fact that over the last 40 years the literature on mental health in the field of assisted reproduction has insisted on the need to be a multidisciplinary and comprehensive field where the patient must be cared for mentally and physically, today mental health is not incorporated as a necessary part of the treatment. Only recently have some private clinics included emotional support units. Finally, the question of what governments are doing to protect patients and their mental health in this field remains a mystery. It is an area where the principle of laissez faire reigns.

Notes

1 Sangomas are legally recognized, under the Traditional Health Practitioners Act of 2007, alongside herbalists, traditional birth attendants, and traditional surgeons.

2 A molar pregnancy is when there is a problem with a fertilized egg, which means a baby and a placenta do not develop the way they should after conception.

References

Agenor, A., & Bhattacharya, S. (2015). Infertility and miscarriage: Common pathways in manifestation and management. *Women's Health, 11*(4), 527–541. https://journals.sagepub.com/doi/pdf/10.2217/WHE.15.19

Allied Market Research. (2021). IVF Services Market Size, Share | IVF Industry Forecast, 2019–2026. www.alliedmarketresearch.com/IVF-in-vitro-fertilization-services-market

Bault, N., & Rusconi, E. (2020). The art of influencing consumer choices: A reflection on recent advances in decision neuroscience. *Frontiers in Psychology, 10*, 3009. www.frontiersin.org/articles/10.3389/fpsyg.2019.03009/full

Bayón, A. (2021). Igenomix ficha a JP Morgan y Morgan Stanley para saltar a la Bolsa de Nueva York a finales de año. *Cinco Días, El País Economía.* March 15. Retrieved from https://cincodias.elpais.com/cincodias/2021/03/12/companias/1615575534_684848.html

Bayón, A., & Martín Simón, P. (2019). El gigante español de la fertilidad IVI ficha a Morgan Stanley para buscar un socio. *Cinco Días, El País*. October 4. Retrieved from https://cincodias.elpais.com/cincodias/2019/10/04/companias/1570213664_146012.html

Bies, R. J., & Tripp, T. M. (2009). Righteous anger: 'Mad as hell' at 'greed is good.' Retrieved from www.porchlightbooks.com/blog/changethis/2009/righteous-anger-mad-as-hell-at-greed-is-good-

Boivin, J., Domar, A. D., Shapiro, D. B., Wischmann, T. H., Fauser, B. C., & Verhaak, C. (2012). Tackling burden in ART: An integrated approach for medical staff. *Human Reproduction (Oxford, England)*, 27(4), 941–950. https://doi.org/10.1093/humrep/der467

Boivin, J., Griffiths, E., & Venetis, C. A. (2011). Emotional distress in infertile women and failure of assisted reproductive technologies: Meta-analysis of prospective psychosocial studies. *British Medical Journal, 342*, 223.

Boivin, J., Scanlan, L. C., & Walker, S. M. (1999). Why are infertile patients not using psychosocial counselling? *Human Reproduction, 14*(5), 1384–1391. https://doi.org/10.1093/humrep/14.5.1384

Bottomley, C., & Bourne, T. (2009). Diagnosing miscarriage. *Best Practice Research Clinic in Obstetric Gynaecology, 23*(4), 463–477. https://pubmed.ncbi.nlm.nih.gov/19502113/

Bravo, P. (2021). KKR entra en fertilidad con la compra de GeneraLife a Investindustrial. *Expansión.* November 10. Retrieved from www.expansion.com/empresas/2021/11/10/618b054e468aeb81328b4667.html

Brody, H. (2010). Professional medical organizations and commercial conflicts of interest: Ethical issues. *Annals of Family Medicine, 8*(4), 354–358. https://doi.org/10.1370/afm.1140

Burgos, J. (2022). Singapore billionaire Peter Lim eyes investment in Spanish fertility firm IVI-RMA amid buyout bids. *Reuters.* March 7. Retrieved from www.forbes.com/sites/jonathanburgos/2022/03/07/singapore-billionaire-peter-lim-eyes-investment-in-spanish-fertility-firm-ivi-rma-amid-buyout-bids/?sh=fceb55486a7c

Cahn, N. R. (2012). The new kinship. *100 Geo. L.J.* 367. Retrieved from https://scholarship.law.gwu.edu/faculty_publications/371/

Casado, R. (2021). La fertilidad mueve más de 4000 millones de euros en operaciones corporativas. *El Economista*. December 11. Retrieved from www.eleconomista.es/empresas-finanzas/noticias/11517077/12/21/La-fertilidad-mueve-mas-de-4000-millones-en-operaciones-corporativas.html

Caulfield, T. (2020). Dr. Oz's hydroxychloroquine advocacy seduces Trump as coronavirus wellness woo surges. NBC News. Timothy Caulfield, Canada Research Chair in Health Law and Policy at the University of Alberta. April 19. Retrieved from www.nbcnews.com/think/opinion/dr-oz-s-hydroxychloroquine-advocacy-seduces-trump-coronavirus-wellness-woo-ncna1185596

CMA. (2022). Competition and markets authority. Fertility clinics' compliance with consumer law: findings published. Government UK. September 23. Retrieved from www.gov.uk/government/news/fertility-clinics-compliance-with-consumer-law-findings-published

CNRHA. (2022). Comisión Nacional de Reproducción Humana Asistida https://cnrha.sanidad.gob.es/miembros/vocales/

Connolly, M. P., Hoorens, S., Chambers, G. M., & ESHRE Reproduction and Society Task Force. (2010). On behalf of the ESHRE Reproduction and Society Task Force, The costs and consequences of assisted reproductive technology: An economic perspective. *Human Reproduction Update, 16*(6), 603–613. https://doi.org/10.1093/humupd/dmq013

Cooper Companies. (2021). Press release. CooperCompanies Completes Acquisition of Generate Life Sciences. San Ramón, California. December 17. Retrieved from https://investor.coopercos.com/news-releases/news-release-details/coopercompanies-completes-acquisition-generate-life-sciencesr?utm_source=gls visto el 25 octubre 2022.

Crawford, G. E., & Ledger, W. L. (2019). In vitro fertilisation/intracytoplasmic sperm injection beyond 2020. BJOG: *International Journal Of Obstetrics & Gynaecology, 126*(2), 237–243. doi: 10.1111/1471-0528.15526

CreateFertility. (2022). CreateFertility. Retrieved from www.createfertility.co.uk/donor-treatments/treatment-with-donor-sperm

Crossley, C. D. (2009). Emotional and behavioral reactions to social undermining: A closer look at perceived offender motives. *Organizational Behavior and Human Decision Processes, 108*, 14–24.

de Castro, M. H. M., Mendonça, C. R., Noll, M., de Abreu Tacon, F. S., & do Amaral, W. N. (2021). Psychosocial aspects of gestational grief in women undergoing infertility treatment: A systematic review of qualitative and quantitative evidence. *International Journal of Environmental Research and Public Health, 18*(24), 13143. https://doi.org/10.3390/ijerph182413143

de Klerk, C., Heijnen, E. M., Macklon, N. S., Duivenvoorden, H. J., Fauser, B. C., Passchier, J., et al. (2006). The psychological impact of IVF failure after two or more cycles of IVF with a mild versus standard treatment strategy. *Human Reproduction, 21*, 721–727.

de la Rochebrochard, E., Soullier, N., Peikrishvili, R., Guibert, J., & Bouyer, J. (2008). High in vitro fertilization discontinuation rate in France. *International Journal of Gynaecology and Obstetrics: The Official Organ of the International Federation of Gynaecology and Obstetrics, 103*(1), 74–75. https://doi.org/10.1016/j.ijgo.2008.05.009

Domar, A. D., Smith, K., Conboy, L., Iannone, M., & Alper, M. (2010). A prospective investigation into the reasons why insured United States patients drop out of in vitro fertilization treatment. *Fertility and Sterility, 94*, 1457–1459.

ESHRE. (2020). ART fact sheet. European Society of Human Reproduction and Embryology. Retrieved from file:///C:/Users/Usuario/Downloads/ESHRE_ARTFactSheet_2022.pdf

Eurostat. (2018). Public employment – Spain. Retrieved from https://ec.europa.eu/eurostat/statistics-explained/index.php?title=Archive:Public_employment_-Spain#:~:text=Statistics%3A%20The%20total%20number%20of,and%2099%20530%20in%20Universities

Fertility Network. (2022). Fertility Network UK. https://fertilitynetworkuk.org/get-involved/our-supporters/

Fresenius. (2020). Investor news. Fresenius Helios acquires fertility services provider Eugin Group. December 21. Retrieved from www.fresenius.com/sites/default/files/2021-11/FSE_Helios_Acquisition_Eugin_e.pdf

Gameiro, S., Verhaak, C. M., Kremer, J. A., & Boivin, J. (2013). Why we should talk about compliance with assisted reproductive technologies (ART): A systematic review and meta-analysis of ART compliance rates. *Human Reproduction Update, 19*(2), 124–135. https://doi.org/10.1093/humupd/dms045

González, A. (2022). Spanish fertility firm IVI-RMA attracts buyout bids worth $2.2 billion. *Reuters*. January 2021. Retrieved from www.reuters.com/article/ivirma-ma-private-equity-idUSL8N2U773O

Goodwin, N., Roach, B., Torras, M., Harris, J., & Nelson, J. (2019). *Principles of Economics in Context*. London: Routledge.

Guerra, D., Llobera, A., Veiga, A., et al. (1998). Psychiatric morbidity in couples attending a fertility service. *Human Reproduction, 13*, 1733–1736.

Hawkins, J. (2013). Selling ART: An empirical assessment of advertising on fertility clinics' websites. *Indiana Law Journal, 88*(4), Article 1. Retrieved from www.repository.law.indiana.edu/ilj/vol88/iss4/1

HFEA. (2022a). Human Fertilisation & Embriology Authority. The HFEA responds to the CMAS report on fertility clinics compliance with consumer law. Retrieved from www.hfea.gov.uk/about-us/news-and-press-releases/2022-news-and-press-releases/the-hfea-responds-to-the-cmas-report-on-fertility-clinics-compliance-with-consumer-law/

HFEA. (2022b). Human Fertilisation & Embryology Authority. About us. Meet our authority members. Retrieved from www.hfea.gov.uk/about-us/our-people/meet-our-authority-members/

Hodgson, L. (2022). As more VC money floods into fertility, some startups are feeling left out (April 26). https://pitchbook.com/news/articles/venture-capital-fertility-technology-femtech

Howard. S. (2018). The hidden costs of infertility treatment. *British Medical Journal,* 361, k2204. doi: https://doi.org/10.1136/bmj.k2204

Hu, L., Du, J., Lv, H., Zhao, J., Chen, M., Wang, Y., et al... (2018). Influencing factors of pregnancy loss and survival probability of clinical pregnancies conceived through assisted reproductive technology. *Reproduction Biology and Endocrinology, 16*, 74. https://doi.org/10.1186/s12958-018-0390-6

IMAP M&A Consultants AG. (2021). Healthcare Industry. Sector: Healthcare services and facilities. 2021 Sector Report. Retrieved from https://southandes.com/content/uploads/imap-healthcare-industry-report.pdf

Immedico. (2023). The benefits of assisted reproduction centers amounted to 570 million in 2022. Immedico Hospitalario. April 20. Retrieved from www.immedicohospitalario.es/noticia/38625/los-beneficios-de-los-centros-de-reproduccion-asistida-ascendieron-a.html

Investors 23andme. (2022). Investor presentation. November 2022. Retrieved from https://investors.23andme.com/static-files/8db681b8-4ea3-452f-a3e6-3a151d8866d9.

Irving, G., Neves, A. L., Dambha-Miller, H., Oishi, A., Tagashira, H., Verho, A., & Holden, J. (2017). International variations in primary care physician consultation time: A systematic review of 67 countries. *BMJ Open, 7*, e017902. doi:10.1136/ bmjopen-2017-017902

IVI. (2023). IVI-RMA is the largest assisted reproduction group in the world. Retrieved from https://ivi-fertility.com/

Karadima, S. (2022). Reproductive tech: A fertile area for investment. August 2. Retrieved from https://medical-technology.nridigital.com/medical_technology_aug22/ivf_reproductive_tech_investment

Kass, N. E. (2001). An ethics framework for public health. *American Journal of Public Health, 91*(11), 1776–1782. https://doi.org/10.2105/ajph.91.11.1776

Kilgore, E. (2022). Mehmet Oz recently flip-flopped to an extreme abortion stance. *Intelligencer*. August 31. Retrieved from https://nymag.com/intelligencer/2022/08/mehmet-oz-just-flip-flopped-to-an-extreme-abortion-stance.html

KKR. (2022). KKR Today. Retrieved from www.kkr.com/kkr-today

Kossoudji, S. A. (2005). The economics of assisted reproduction. Institute for the Study of Labor (IZA). *Discussion Paper No. 1458* January. Deutsche Post World Net. & the University of Bonn. Retrieved from https://docs.iza.org/dp1458.pdf

Krawiec, K. D. (2009). Altruism and intermediation in the market for babies. *Washington and Lee Law Review, 66*(1)(203), 213–214. https://scholarlycommons.law.wlu.edu/wlulr/vol66/iss1/5/

Kuhnt, A. K., & Passet-Wittig, J. (2022). Families formed through assisted reproductive technology: Causes, experiences, and consequences in an international context. *Reproductive Biomedicine & Society Online, 14*, 289–296. https://doi.org/10.1016/j.rbms.2022.01.001

Lancastle, D., & Boivin, J. (2008). A feasibility study of a brief coping intervention (PRCI) for the waiting period before a pregnancy test during fertility treatment. *Human Reproduction, 23*, 2299–2307.

Lukse, M. P., & Vacc, N. A. (1999). Grief, depression, and coping in women undergoing infertility treatment. *Obstetrics & Gynecology, 93*(2), 245–251. www.sciencedirect.com/science/article/abs/pii/S0029784498004323?via%3Dihub

Matthiesen, S. M. S., Frederiksen, Y., Ingerslev, H. J., & Zachariae, R. (2011). Stress, distress, and outcome of assisted reproductive technology (ART): A meta-analysis. *Human Reproduction, 26*, 2763–2776.

McDowell, S., & Murray, A. (2011). Barriers to continuing in vitro fertilisation – Why do patients exit fertility treatment? *The Australian & New Zealand Journal of Obstetrics & Gynaecology, 51*(1), 84–90. https://doi.org/10.1111/j.1479-828X.2010.01236.x

Miller, L. M., Wallace, G., Birdsall, M. A., Hammond, E. R., & Peek, J. C. (2021). Dropout rate and cumulative birth outcomes in couples undergoing in vitro fertilization within a funded and actively managed system of care in New Zealand. *Fertility and Sterility, 116*(1), 114–122. https://doi.org/10.1016/j.fertnstert.2021.01.041

Morgan Stanley. (2022). Earnings release. Retrieved from www.morganstanley.com/about-us-ir/shareholder/2q2022.pdf

National Lottery Funding. (2022). Community Fund. Retrieved from www.tnlcommunityfund.org.uk/about

Pasch, L. A., Gregorich, S. E., Katz, P. K., Millstein, S. G., Nachtigall, R. D., Bleil, M. E., & Adler, N. E. (2012). Psychological distress and in vitro fertilization outcome. *Fertility and Sterility, 98*(2), 459–464. https://doi.org/10.1016/j.fertnstert.2012.05.023

Pasch, L. A., Holley, S. R., Bleil, M. E., Shehab, D., Katz, P. P., & Adler, N. E. (2016). Addressing the needs of fertility treatment patients and their partners: Are they informed of and do they receive mental health services? *Fertility and Sterility, 106*(1), 209–215. https://doi.org/10.1016/j.fertnstert.2016.03.006

Patrizio, P., Albertini, D. F., Gleicher, N., & Caplan, A. (2022). The changing world of IVF: The pros and cons of new business models offering assisted reproductive technologies. *Journal of Assisted Reproduction and Genetics, 39*(2), 305–313. https://doi.org/10.1007/s10815-022-02399-y

Quirón Salud. (2022). Prueba de Fertilidad – Reserva Ovárica, 38€. Retrieved from https://e-quironsalud.es/estudios-geneticos/128-prueba-de-fertilidad-reserva-ovarica?gclid=Cj0KCQiA99ybBhD9ARIsALvZavVnGRyzRqAwKch5LknEBVX0HxYMFCgomByohqr7duZfm7eCN8tFvUIaAj78EALw_wcB

Reardon, D. C. (2018). The abortion and mental health controversy: A comprehensive literature review of common ground agreements, disagreements, actionable recommendations, and research opportunities. *SAGE Open Medicine, 6*, 2050312118807624. https://doi.org/10.1177/2050312118807624

Robbins, R. (2017). Investors see big money in infertility. And they're transforming the industry. *STAT. Reporting from the frontiers of health and medicine*. Boston Globe Media USA. December 4. Retrieved from www.statnews.com/2017/12/04/infertility-industry-investment/

Sage, W. M. (1999). Regulating through information: Disclosure laws and American health care. *Columbia Law Review, 99*(7), 1701–1829. https://doi.org/10.2307/1123624

Sagili, H., & Divers, M. (2011). Modern management of miscarriage. *The Obstetrician & Gynaecologist, 9*(2), 102–108. https://obgyn.onlinelibrary.wiley.com/doi/abs/10.1576/toag.9.2.102.27311

Schröder, A. K., Katalinic, A., Diedrich, K., & Ludwig, M. (2004). Cumulative pregnancy rates and drop-out rates in a German IVF programme: 4102 cycles in 2130 patients. *Reproductive Biomedicine Online, 8*(5), 600–606. https://doi.org/10.1016/s1472-6483(10)61110-8

Terry, M. (2016). Meet the $200 million startup that unwinds a woman's biological clock. *BioSpace*. Retrieved from www.biospace.com/article/meet-the-200-million-startup-that-unwinds-a-woman-s-biological-clock-b-dr-oz-b-joins-board-/

TFP. (2022). TFP Fertility. Retrieved from https://tfp-fertility.com

The Economist. (2019). The fertility business is booming. August 8. Retrieved from www.economist.com/business/2019/08/08/the-fertility-business-is-booming?

Troude, P., Guibert, J., Bouyer, J., de La Rochebrochard, E., & DAIFI Group. (2014). Medical factors associated with early IVF discontinuation. *Reproductive Biomedicine Online, 28*(3), 321–329. https://doi.org/10.1016/j.rbmo.2013.10.018

Tushnet, R., & Goldman, E. (2014). *Advertising & marketing law: Cases and materials*. CreateSpace Independent Publishing Platform.

University of Pittsburgh Medical Center. (2021). Women's health. Egg freezing age limit: Why age matters. Affiliated with the University of Pittsburgh Schools of the Health Sciences. April 16. Retrieved from https://share.upmc.com/2021/04/egg-freezing-age-limit/

Verhaak, C. M., Smeenk, J. M., van Minnen, A., Kremer, J. A., & Kraaimaat, F. W. (2005). A longitudinal, prospective study on emotional adjustment before, during and after consecutive fertility treatment cycles. *Human Reproduction, 20*(8), 2253–2260. https://doi.org/10.1093/humrep/dei015

Verhaak, C. M., Smeenk, J. M. J., Nahuis, M. J., Kremer, J. A. M., Braat, D. D. M. (2007). Long-term psychological adjustment to IVF/ICSI treatment in women. *Human Reproduction, 22*(1), 305–308. https://doi.org/10.1093/humrep/del355

Web Capital Riesgo. (2022). KKR adquiere IVI-RMA en una operación valorada en €3.000 millones. March 29. Retrieved from www.webcapitalriesgo.com/kkr-adquiere-ivi-rma-en-una-operacion-valorada-en-e3-000-millones/

Weller, C. (2017). What you need to know about egg-freezing, the hot new perk at Google, Apple, and Facebook. *Business Insider*. September 17. Retrieved from www.businessinsider.com/egg-freezing-at-facebook-apple-google-hot-new-perk-2017-9

Zareba, K., La Rosa, V. L., Ciebiera, M., Makara-Studzińska, Commodari, K. E., & Gierus, J. (2020). Psychological effects of abortion. An updated narrative review. *Eastern Journal of Medicine, 25*(3), 477–483. https://jag.journalagent.com/ejm/pdfs/EJM_25_3_477_483.pdf

4 Reproductive agency and ART

The role of hospitals, legal frameworks, and the media

Introduction

By way of an overview and to approach the phenomenon of women who have chosen to become mothers on their own through assisted reproductive technology, I will examine the process that begins when women decide to undergo treatment with assisted reproductive techniques in private clinics (having been denied access to ART in public hospitals), how they handle the treatment, how they imagine their gestation and childbirth, their descriptions of giving birth in public hospitals, and the treatment that the obstetric teams give them. All the participants declared that they had felt empowered when they took the following decisions: (a) becoming a mother; (b) choosing a private clinic to receive treatment; (c) selecting (where possible) the donor(s) of genetic material; (d) attempting to manage assisted reproduction treatment; (e) choosing a highly rated public hospital; (f) drawing up a birth plan; and (g) selecting a doula or a companion to be with them during this process and in the hospital. However, their empowerment – which the participants understand to be their capacity to control their own lives, to exercise their rights, and take strategic decisions in terms of their own reproductive health – was nullified when they were in labor and the puerperium in the hospitals.

They reported that their birth plans were not taken into consideration. They suffered dehumanizing treatment at the hands of the medical teams which constituted obstetric violence in not informing them about the effects of the medication administered to induce labor, compelling them to have a cesarean regardless of their explicit wish not to, and neither caring for nor accompanying the women in labor. I am aware that there are parts of this process, such as the independent decision to become mothers using ART and donated genetic material, which are specific to these women. Nonetheless, there are other parts of the process, such as the treatment received from the obstetric teams, that can be applied to all those women who give birth in hospitals, regardless of their age, whether they have a partner or not, or whether they used ART. Whatever the case, the sociocultural construction of mothers' age and of choosing a non-normative family with the help of ART, condition and bias the perception of this population in the legislative, medical, social, and media spheres. This will be the focus of the analysis given further. One of my aims in this ethnographic study is to illuminate how becoming mothers by choice

DOI: 10.4324/9781003269755-5

may be empowering and a site of social change for women who resist replicating "conventional" forms of motherhood. In the next section, I will contextualize reproductive politics, access to ART, and the inequities participants confronted.

Natural pregnancy, age, "solo" mothers, earning power, and ART

Do "solo" women aged 35 and above "deserve" to become mothers with the help of ART? Moreover, are they entitled to access ART with public funds under the National Health System (NHS)? Is it "natural" to become a mother after the age of 35? One of my purposes in this section is to deconstruct the idea of whether it is "natural" for women to procreate after the age of 35, and the label of "advanced age" of women in order to get pregnant. These issues are relevant in the sociocultural, medical, and media perception of this population. Why is the age of women important, or their decision to become mothers on their own with ART using public funds? The perception of society, including medical teams and legislators or the media, has an influence on who gains access or not to ART in the NHS. For example, in Austria only married heterosexual couples are permitted access to ART (Präg & Mills, 2017). This perception also affects the treatment and the type of childbirth that the obstetric teams suggest for, or impose on, these women in public hospitals in both Spain and the United Kingdom, as will be shown further.

First of all, what is "natural"? Singer and Wells (1983, p. 193) explain: "Whether a certain practice is natural depends on one's philosophical conception of human nature. Two views can be distinguished: a) the descriptive view is that what is natural occurs in nature untouched by human intervention". Consequently, ART is unnatural and so is medicine. On the other hand, the teleological view looks to human ends. By this account, since ART and "medicine involve the exercise of human capacities, they are perfectly natural" (Singer, 1983, p. 193). The argument against older women's childbearing based on the perception that it goes "against nature" disregards the fact that nowadays in the Global North it is socially and medically acceptable to create a temporary or permanent "against nature" non-fertile state in women with the use of contraceptives or surgery. It is also regarded appropriate for menopausal women to confront nature by using hormone replacement therapy to defer the consequences of the menopause (Peterson, 2005) or to vaccinate 12-year-old girls against human papilloma virus to help protect them against various cancers. It is also accepted that men have vasectomies, use condoms, take Viagra, and, in general, that sexually active individuals may use barrier methods to prevent venereal diseases.

Second, women's age is important for the NHS in the United Kingdom and in Spain. Both services discriminate against women who are 35 years and older and who want to access fertility treatment, who may face waiting lists for ART in both countries that may take up to three years. Yet, the medical fact remains that the pregnancy success rate is most strongly correlated with the age of the ova, donated or otherwise. Age becomes an issue in these women's lives: (a) they do not have access to public fertility treatment if they are older than 35 years; (b) the terms used to categorize them as pregnant women are ageist; and (c) obstetric teams take decisions regarding the type of childbirth women will have depending on their chronological age, not biological age, nor ova age, which in half of the sample reported here was donated from women in their early twenties. The terms used to refer to women's pregnancy when they are aged 35 or older are: "advanced maternal age" or "geriatric pregnancy" in English-speaking countries, and "añosa", which is employed in Spanish-speaking countries and means "aged woman". To label the gestation of these women with those expressions is ageist in both languages and denotes sociocultural constructions of pregnant women aged 35 and above as "old". Indeed women's use of ART has exposed age prejudices associated with women.

Petropanagos (2015) argues that pregnancy at an "advanced maternal age" may be perceived as violating social norms surrounding motherhood, where the "good" mother is construed as young, active, and self-sacrificing. However, moral criticisms of women aged 35 or older rely on a particular conception of motherhood that is, possibly, ageist and sexist, relying on restricted notions of the family. The allegation that women who become mothers in their late thirties and older might not have the energy to cope with babies and teenagers contradicts the fact that older women play, and have played historically, a key role in childrearing, including being the sole or main carer for their children and grandchildren. Moreover, ageism tends to reinforce social inequalities as it is more pronounced towards older women (Ayalon and Tesch-Römer, 2017). Intersectional identities can result in a cumulative negative impact for older women who choose to become mothers on their own as they already have a history of disrespectful treatment for other reasons: sexism, bias against solo mothers, sexual orientation, racism, and disability. Some reasons for rejecting an upper age limit are linked to this critique of motherhood. Furthermore, age limits are sexist because no comparable age limits exist for men. Men are not condemned for becoming fathers in their late thirties, forties, fifties, or older, which is a regular event. "It's also hard to make an upper limit because it contradicts reproductive liberties", says Jeffrey Kahn director of the Johns Hopkins Berman Institute of Bioethics, adding that it would be unfair to restrict women from receiving fertility treatments when men can procreate "well into their 70s" (Richards, 2015).

Additionally, although the average age of menopause remains around 52, life expectancy has increased dramatically over the last century, more so for women than for men. It is also a fact that women have given birth to babies naturally in their forties and fifties prior to the advent of ART services. Eijkemans et al. (2014) state that demographers use the 17th, 18th, and 19th centuries to determine what happened in so-called natural fertility populations, which lacked access to birth control and family planning. In all these populations, the average age at last birth ranges from 39 to 42 years. Becoming a mother beyond 35 years of age is not abnormal. Reproductive endocrinologists Steiner and Paulson suggest that: "There is no reason to say women in their 50s cannot be good mothers". Their research compares women who gave birth after 50 to younger mothers in their forties and thirties and concluded that: "our data do not support the hypothesis that mothers of advanced maternal age have reduced parenting capacity due to physical or mental ability or parenting stress" (2007, p. 1332). The data suggest that patients up to the age of 55 who are carefully selected and well managed can have safe pregnancies. Another study in Denmark of women aged between 20 and 40 years states that most women labelled as of "advanced maternal age" have healthy pregnancies, especially if they begin pregnancy in good health and seek prompt prenatal care (Rothman et al., 2014). In addition, there is a difference between chronological and biological age. Chronological age refers to the number of years a person has been alive, biological age takes many lifestyle factors into consideration, including diet and nutrition, exercise and sleeping habits, stress, mental and emotional health, exposure to environmental and other toxins, and chronic conditions, to name but a few. Biological age is a better measure of aging and how healthy a person is. However, the mechanisms underlying age-related DNA methylation changes remain mostly undiscovered (Ciccarone et al., 2018). These facts indicate that concerns about whether older women will survive long enough to care for their children are unsubstantiated.

Third, delaying childbirth substantially boosts women's earning power. Women who give birth in their late thirties and early forties also tend to live longer, and their children score higher on tests of cognitive ability than children born to women in their twenties. Many older women report feeling more emotionally and financially prepared for parenting. Goises et al. (2017) conducted a study of three UK birth cohorts that shows the association between advanced maternal age and higher child cognitive ability. The trend all over the developed world in recent years has been more women having more children later; and whether it is a first child or a later child, more women giving birth are 35 and older, which is still classified as "advanced maternal age", and children born to the 35- to 39-year-olds did significantly better in cognitive testing than children born to the younger mothers. According to Goisis et al. (2017), older mothers were more likely to be educated and socioeconomically better off. "These women tend to be advantaged", and to take better care of themselves during pregnancy.

Fourth, according to Schenker (2011), legal prohibitions or undue limitations on individuals availing themselves of ART services can be claimed to violate the rights to have a family and to reproductive health. The World Medical Association's Statement on ART, adopted by its General Assembly in October 2006, observes that "inability to become a parent without medical intervention (…) is a cause of major psychological illness and its treatment is clearly medical". ART treatment is undoubtedly justified as medical service and medical attention assisting achievement of the goal of reproductive health. Its prohibition or undue obstruction is a human rights violation (Shencker 2011, p. 27). Donor egg technology makes conception possible at later ages and it may contribute to a wider societal process of reconsidering women's age markers by making biological indicators such as the menopause and age less relevant as social markers (Becker 2000). Issues raised in the debate about access to ARTs and women's age are intimately intertwined with other debates, such as those to do with feminism, women's education and earning power, reproductive agency, reproductive politics, and public health policy.

"I would have done a handstand with my ears in order to get myself pregnant!"

I explain in this section how the participants experience assisted reproduction treatments to reverse the limits imposed by biology. The intense desire to get pregnant meant being aware of the need to adapt and undergo ART in the best possible way, thus freeing themselves from the biological restriction involved in the lack of sperm, their oocytes' limited number, or the poor quality of their eggs. For these women, ART meant reproductive freedom in several key ways, seeking to preserve fertility against the effects of time, and having access to sperm and egg donors. The women who had chosen egg freezing felt empowered because this was a way to preserve oocytes against the threat of age, disease, or early menopause. ART expanded fertility options for these women, who had invested time in their education: all of them had university degrees and some postgraduate studies. Reproductive technologies also gave them the chance to strengthen their professional careers. Therefore resorting to ART was, in all the cases, driven by their own pervasive desire for children; and by rescheduling biological motherhood to a later time, it enabled them to establish a career, and in one case to undergo cancer treatment with less of a risk of missing out on biological motherhood. From this perspective, the desire to have a child is more important than any accompanying feeling of alienation or physical discomfort in the reproductive treatment, or private clinics' profits, taking into account that all the participants were able to afford their treatments. The cost per live birth is highest in the United Kingdom (35.647€) and lowest in Spain (21.489€) (Crawford et al., 2016).

For example, Sara, 40 years old, a Spanish economist who lives in Spain, and who got pregnant two years ago with the help of an anonymous sperm donor at a private clinic, gave birth at a public hospital and remarks about her treatment:

> Something that worried me during my treatment was preparing the medication and self-administering it ... But I would have done a handstand with my ears in order to get myself pregnant! [she laughs] And thanks to ART my dream became reality.

The fear of doing it wrong and thinking that they might mess up the whole process means that the administering of the medication entails added stress to the assisted reproductive treatment. The women have to do it exactly as it is explained to them in the clinic, taking care not to inject an inferior dose or to do it incorrectly, reading the directions for use, preparing it calmly and checking it to avoid mistakes. Another participant is Thelma, 39 years of age, British, from London and who works for an NGO, gave birth to her baby two months ago using her own eggs and a non-anonymous sperm donor from a Danish sperm bank. She was treated at a private clinic in London and this is how she described her treatment:

> I wasn't looking forward to injecting myself every day and so I thought, "Right, I'll make it nice. I kept the ritual of lighting a candle every evening. I found the

whole process incredibly empowering and positive … I was taking control of my life".

For most of them, the treatment involved using symbolic rituals such as lighting candles before injecting the hormones or visualizing their body pregnant with the creation of vision boards, which included photographs of bellies in an advanced stage of gestation so as to imagine and make real through images their pregnant body. This is how Rosa, a 52-year-old Spanish architect who had her child at the age of 46 in a public hospital in Madrid, having received anonymous egg and sperm donation at a private clinic in Spain, explains it:

> I so wanted to have a baby that I prepared myself mentally by projecting my vision of it: I printed pictures from the internet of the bellies of pregnant women, of newly born babies, and I stuck them on a card, and I would look at them every day, imagining that it could be my belly and that it could be my baby. Truly, ART gave me the chance to be a mother. Injecting myself and taking lots of medication every day was secondary compared to the wish to become a mother. And so I chose to create the physical possibility through medication and the mental possibility through my desire and imagination to have a baby.

The symbolic rituals, a healthy diet, taking physical exercise, and visualizing their pregnancy was daily practice in the lives of these women, which fed their hope that the assisted reproductive treatment would prove to be successful. For those women who, because of their age or because the treatment did not work with their own eggs, as was the case for Eva, who had frozen her eggs when she was 39 and when 43 she used them but they failed to result in any embryo, the only option left is that of egg donation. For Eva, a doctor in biology and resident in Spain, the fact that no viable embryo was produced with her eggs meant going through what the literature in psychology calls genetic grief (García-Lumbreras, 2019), the process of sadness that some women go through when they learn the news that they will not be able to use their eggs to conceive their baby. Nevertheless, Eva became pregnant at the first attempt with anonymous egg and sperm donation at age of 44:

> I was very hopeful, thinking that as I had frozen my eggs when I was 39 years old, I had a good chance of getting pregnant with my own eggs and with the sperm of the man who was then my partner, I was 43. However, the embryos they implanted in me did not lead to a pregnancy. I was left terribly sad. Not long after I broke up with my partner and went to a clinic, where they offered me the possibility of anonymous egg and sperm donation. My desire to be a mother was so strong that I said yes. The clinic psychologist helped me to overcome both bereavements: the genetic, which I did not know that this type of grief existed but she called it that; and that of having broken up with a partner, whom, I realised, I was only with in order to create a family. When I had my baby in my arms I felt that everything that I had done had been absolutely worth it.

Thus, beyond the genetic material, according to the participants, the team of professionals working at the private assisted reproduction clinics advised focusing on the final objective, which was having a baby, the reasons for which the women wanted to undertake the journey to motherhood and all the positive feelings that the arrival of their child inspired in them. In this way, they managed to find hope again after failed attempts with their own eggs and it is then that they found themselves ready to begin with the option of egg donation. Furthermore, the private clinics informed them that recent studies demonstrated that the mother is able to genetically modify the embryo's gene expression in the first weeks of gestation, in a process explained by "epigenetics" (Huntriss, 2018; O'Neill, 2015). ART opened up the possibility of childbearing to this group of women who wanted to have children on their own and who did not have this option before. Therefore it contributed to empowering these women, granting them more control over their body, reproduction, and motherhood. The following section will deal with participants' plans for a natural birth in hospitals which resulted in another type of delivery marked by medical intervention.

Women's disempowerment: confronting hospital reality, mode of delivery, and its relation with "advanced maternal age" and ART

In this section, the experiences of labor in public hospitals both in Spain and in the United Kingdom will be examined. Most interviewees except one wanted the most natural childbirth possible, that is, a vaginal birth without an induction or cesarean. Most accepted that if the pain was very intense, they would request an epidural, but this was the only intervention that they considered. Two of the participants, living in London, wished to have their baby in a pool designed for this purpose. Most of the participants resident in London had medically recommended cesareans on the basis of their age (35–47 years), and the assisted reproductive treatment. This was despite the fact that in half of the cases, the pregnancy had been achieved using the donation of sperm and eggs from donors in their early twenties, and that only two of the interviewees had any prior medical condition.

All of the women said that they led a healthy lifestyle and had no problems during gestation. All the participants in Spain were given epidural injections, in most cases labor was induced, and in a minority of cases a caesarean was performed. Vicky, 46 years old, a mental health nurse from Eastern Europe, who has been living in London for the past 23 years, had given birth to her baby three weeks prior to our interview. She had been treated at a private clinic in Spain using anonymous egg and sperm donors in their early twenties, and became pregnant at her first attempt. She gave birth at a public hospital in London and talks about her experience:

> I really wanted a water birth at home and I hired a pool. I had a very gentle beginning but then it wasn't progressing enough. I ended up in a hospital and had an emergency caesarean. I was so shivery on the operating table, it was just such a nightmare, I've never had any operations in my life, and I never expected this. The doctors knew that I had IVF, that the baby was conceived with a double

> donation, with donors in their twenties. Nevertheless, they put me automatically in a high-risk category because of my age and because of IVF, but I never had any medical condition! They didn't know how to deal with it. They thought that things might get complicated. I didn't have any complications during pregnancy … If I had been in a calm and proper state, I would have never agreed to a caesarean, I really thought that the caesarean would have been such a last resort. I thought that if I went to hospital, at least they'd give me an injection to numb my pain, and then I could continue pushing, but they wouldn't let me go into the pool at all. They had just attached the machines on my belly, they had to monitor me continuously … they told me I'd have to be in a hospital, on the labor ward. And I was, like, "Well, I'm actually choosing home birth, you know?" I was so confident that I could trust my body, and it would happen, but it just stopped … I tried to push after they gave me synthetic oxytocin and an epidural, and I was just feeling so horrible with all this, because I really was just completely medicated when I wanted it to be so natural …

Vicky is grateful for the work of her doula, which made up for the lack of obstetric personnel who neither accompanied nor cared for her during the process. She emphasizes the apparent ignorance of the obstetric team and their hostility. The medical team did not take into account that (a) she had no medical condition, (b) she had a problem-free gestation, and (c) the ovum and sperm were from young donors. The obstetrician only focused on her chronological age and the use of ART, classifying her case as high risk, despite the fact that the research suggests that the mother's overall health (biological age) is more important than chronological age per se (Ciccarone et al., 2018; Kitzinger, 2011), and that the quality of donated eggs from women in their twenties with proven fertility are key for a successful pregnancy (American Society for Reproductive Medicine, 2012). Thus, the actions of the medical team show their prejudice against the age of the participant, imposing a caesarean upon her, which caused Vicky to lose her calm and submit, to her regret, to the judgement of the specialist.

A review of 26 studies that provided data from 17 countries, involving more than 15,000 women in a wide range of settings and circumstances showed that: "Women who received continuous labor support may be more likely to give birth 'spontaneously', i.e. give birth vaginally. In addition, women may be less likely to use pain medications, and may be more likely to be satisfied and have shorter labors" (Bohren et al., 2017). On the other hand, a series of studies published in the *Lancet* (Boerma et al., 2018) found that the use of cesarean sections is rising rapidly worldwide with experts saying the procedure is growing at an "alarming" rate. The World Health Organization estimates that around 10%–15% of births require a C-section due to complications and it has suggested that rates higher than that are excessive (WHO, 2018). The research found that the procedure is overused in rich countries. The global increase in its prevalence has been attributed to more women giving birth in medical institutions like hospitals where the procedure is implemented more often. According to the OECD (2017), in the United Kingdom the rate of cesareans was 27.4%, while in Spain it was 24.4%. Nevertheless, the cesarean delivery rate increases in direct proportion to age in both countries: Hospital Episodes Statistics (HES) containing records of all patients admitted to NHS hospitals in England show that 35% of cesareans were performed in women aged 30–39 years, and 45% in women aged 40 and onwards (HES, 2018). And the National Institute of Statistics in Spain indicate that 30% of cesareans were performed in women aged 35–39 years; and 39% in women aged 40–44 years, and 58% in women aged 45–49 years (INE, 2015).

Fay, a 50-year-old British head of research at a private company in London, gave birth to her son at the age of 47 years. She had been treated at a private clinic in London with sperm donor from a US sperm bank and her sister's eggs. She describes how she ended up having a cesarean at a London public hospital:

> My pregnancy could not have been better. I wasn't sick once, it was amazing. The combination of being a first-time mother at 47 years old and IVF made me in the doctors' mind high risk, so I had a C-section.

Gabrielle, 48 years of age, a British university graduate who owns her own company and lives in London, was treated three years ago at a private clinic in Spain with anonymous egg and sperm donation, from donors in their early twenties. She explains why she had a C-section at a London public hospital:

> I was planning to give birth naturally although this hospital has a policy that every woman over 40 has to be induced. I was 45 … what frustrated me was that I had a textbook pregnancy. I didn't have anything untoward, so they started the process of inducing me and it wasn't working so I had a C-section.

A study published in the *Canadian Medical Association Journal* (Korb et al., 2019) suggests that the trade-off of risk versus convenience of scheduled C-sections for women aged 35 years and older is dramatically skewed. Researchers found that cesarean delivery is associated with a higher risk of severe acute maternal morbidity than vaginal delivery. They also found that women over 35 years who had planned C-sections were at greater risk for a range of severe maternal morbidities, including: hemorrhage, stroke, blood clots in the lungs, kidney, liver and cardiac dysfunction, and admittance to the intensive care unit. Their finding raises questions about the practices of some obstetricians who consider cesarean deliveries to be indicated by "advanced maternal age", with the idea that there will probably be no further pregnancies. Nevertheless, this practice may unnecessarily expose women older than 35 years to the excess risk of severe acute maternal morbidity. Horsager-Boehrer (2019), Head of Obstetrics and Gynecology at the University of Texas, claims that spontaneous labor is the safest route for most patients and their babies. According to WHO (2018, p. 4): "In high-income countries, the proportion of infants delivered at term following induction of labor can be as high as one in four births". Nevertheless, WHO does not recommend induction of labor for women with an uncomplicated pregnancy at gestational age less than 41 weeks, and "the potential need for induction of labor for women with a post-term pregnancy should be discussed with women in advance, so that they have an opportunity to ask questions and understand the benefits and possible risks" (WHO, 2018, p. 5).

Hospitals and obstetric violence

In this section I will analyze the experiences of participants and also my own experience of labor induction. Two of the participants in the present study epitomize the experiences of the majority of the interviewees. They comment on how, despite wishing for a natural birth, they were induced in hospitals. Induction of labor is a practice on which WHO recommends not to exceed the 10% rate. The European Perinatal Health Report (2013, p. 92) states that in the case of the region of Valencia (Spain) there is a 32% of labor inductions in public hospitals, the report does not offer data for the rest of regions in Spain and in the case of England the induction of labor occurs in 21% of cases, however the report does not specify women's age in any region.

Maya, 40 years, British, works for an NGO in London, and was treated at a private clinic in London. After two miscarriages she became pregnant with sperm from a donor and gave birth one year ago at a public hospital in London:

> I know the NHS people pressure women into induction or caesarean if they're older and they had IVF. They induced me. … they loaded me up with drugs and gave me the epidural.

Zoe, a 47-year-old South African living in London, was treated at a private clinic in Spain with an anonymous double (egg and sperm) donation, and gave birth three years ago at a public hospital in London:

> This Hospital has a policy where after the age of 40 they induce you. I didn't really want to be induced but I had no chance.

In my own case, I had my daughter on my own through ART and donated genetic material at the age of 45 years in a private clinic and I gave birth in a public hospital in Madrid. I chose the public hospital "12 de Octubre" because in 2011 it was the first to be awarded the accreditation for the promotion of natural birth, the health of the newborn, and maternal breastfeeding. The Baby Friendly Hospital Initiative is an internationally recognized accreditation created by WHO and UNICEF to encourage hospitals to adopt practices that protect and facilitate exclusive maternal breastfeeding from birth and skin-to-skin contact in order to enable the creation of a bond between mother and child. The "12 de Octubre" hospital stood out as one of the most respectful with the woman and her baby in childbirth. I had consciously prepared myself, researched and weighed up the pros and cons of giving birth depending on which hospital: I joined forums where they discussed which hospitals had the best obstetric services, those that respected the woman's decision to have a "natural" birth the most. When my waters broke, at six o'clock in the morning,

I called the hospital and they told me I had to get there as soon as possible. I arrived with my "Birth Plan" document and gave it to the nurse who told me that I had to wait, and that I could walk along the corridor so that the movement might cause me to start contractions and thus not have to wait long. They told me that if, 12 hours after the waters breaking, labor had not started, they would induce it. The birth plan that I had drawn up in such detail was falling apart before my eyes, without anybody commenting. I remembered a piece of data from the WHO, which asserted that it was not necessary to induce labor before 24 hours after the waters break, and I also bore in mind that a few days before, a hospital nurse had conducted a vaginal examination on me, which I believe might have caused the waters to break before time. They had not informed me of the possible consequences of performing a manual vaginal examination, such as a possible infection or causing the onset of labor (Downe et al., 2013).

And so I found myself walking up and down a corridor. They did not allow me to leave the hospital as they had to monitor me, and the 12 hours passed. The nurse told me that they had to induce labor. I did not want them to, preferring that the baby would come out when she had to come out. I asked to speak with the head of the obstetrics department, who told me that it was necessary to follow the hospital protocol of 12 hours. When I insisted that the WHO stipulated waiting 24 hours, he accepted the negotiation and said that we would wait 24 hours but if I was not in labor by then, I would be induced. I felt hopeful, I had won a small battle. Nevertheless, after 24 hours I was still not in labor. Not allowing me to negotiate for more time, they administered prostaglandin and oxytocin. The nurse had informed me that I would sleep all night and would probably give birth in the morning. So I lay down on the bed as ordered, as they had to monitor the fetus, with many cables connecting my belly to a device. I started to feel sharp, intense cramping pains, which exploded inside me in all directions. I began to have diarrhea, to try to vomit with an empty stomach, my body shook so much that when I went to the bathroom I could not sit on the toilet, writhing uncontrollably. I felt intense cold, I had a fever, I felt very ill, with terrifying pains and stomach cramps. I told the nurses but they were busy. Nobody took care of what was happening to me and hours passed like this. Clearly, the hospital was not following WHO recommendations that assert: "Induction of labor should be performed with caution since the procedure carries the risk of uterine hyperstimulation and rupture, and foetal distress". Or that: "Women receiving oxytocin, misoprostol or other prostaglandins should never be left unattended" (WHO, 2018, p. 7).

Nobody had informed me of the consequences of taking prostaglandin and oxytocin, of their effects on my body. Not one healthcare professional accompanied me at any time. After hours of intense pain, stomach cramps, shaking, diarrhea, and vomiting (caused by complications associated with the use of oxytocin and prostaglandin), they transferred me to the ward next to the delivery room. I had wrapped myself in a blanket because I felt very cold, I was shaking and could not manage to sit down on the bed. A nurse watched me from the doorway and ordered me to sit down on the bed, to take off the blanket, that these were hospital rules, as though

I were purposefully disobeying her orders. Not once did she help me, she only gave me orders. I felt utterly sick. I stared at her and asked her: Do you know what empathy is? Can't you see the state I'm in? In response, she told me that the rules were that I sit on the bed and take off the blanket, and she left the room.

She did not help me, she did nothing other than speak to me of rules while my body was beset by side effects from the hormones, about which nobody had bothered to inform me. Hence the nurse hid behind hospital rules, transferring her responsibility and her negligence to the institution, reaffirming the normative relations of power and repressing behavior that threatened the established hospital protocols. I tried to lie down on the bed, shaking, cold from head to foot. I had far surpassed my pain threshold, so they gave me an epidural, which only had an effect on the left side of my body, which felt dead. The right side was absolutely trembling with pain. When I asked the nurses to correct the unequal result of the epidural on my body, they told me that the anesthetist was very busy. Thirty-two hours after my waters broke, I gave birth. One of the midwives who assisted in my labor told me knowingly that I had been lucky: "you got an obstetrician who favours a humane delivery, if you had got another they would have cut you up". In other words, they would have performed an episiotomy on me. They had placed my daughter in my lap and I felt relieved and overcome with joy, in spite of that statement.

The very morning that I gave birth I was visited by a nurse, when I commented to her that I was producing no breast milk, she suddenly squeezed my nipple roughly, without a word of warning, as if my breast were a cow's udder to milk. After 32 hours of trying to give birth, of the adverse effects of the labor induction hormones, that this nurse should cause me even more pain horrified me. She did not speak to me, she did not ask for permission, she did not warn me of what she was going to do; she treated me as if I were an inanimate object. She probably did not know that "synthetic oxytocin given during labor can negatively affect breastfeeding" (Gomes et al., 2018). I wrote two letters of complaint concerning the treatment I received during my time in the hospital, but never received a reply.

Both neglect of care of the nurse during labor and the omission or concealment of information by the medical team concerning the possible adverse effects of labor induction or of a cesarean, interfere in the decision-making capacity of the woman and constitute "obstetric violence" (Tribunal de Justicia, 2006). This affects women's experiences of childbirth and puerperium in hospitals, resulting in feelings of powerlessness and anxiety. Negative interpersonal relations between caregivers and women in labor have been found to be features of traumatic birth experiences (Elmir et al., 2010). Laws on obstetric violence originate from Venezuela and Argentina, but they are an exception despite the predominance of obstetric violence worldwide. In 2006, Venezuela became the first country to legally define obstetric violence and to classify it as a crime:

> The appropriation of the body and reproductive processes of women by health professionals, which is expressed in dehumanizing treatment, in an abuse of medicalization and pathologization of natural processes, resulting in loss of

> autonomy and ability to freely decide on their bodies and sexuality, negatively impacting the quality of life of women.
>
> (Tribunal de Justicia, 2006, p. 30)

Regarding obstetric violence in the United Kingdom, drawing on wide-ranging evidence and in consultation with women and their families, as well as an ample variety of stakeholders including NHS staff and independent experts, the NHS England commissioned a review chaired by Baroness Julia Cumberlege, who argues:

> We heard that many women are not being offered real choice in the services they can access, and are too often being told what to do, rather than being given information to make their own decisions. We found almost total unanimity from mothers that they want their midwife to be with them from the start, through pregnancy, birth and then after birth. Time and again mothers said that they hardly ever saw the same professional twice. That is unacceptable, inefficient and must change. We spend £560 million each year on compensating families for negligence during maternity care. And when things do go wrong, the fear of litigation can prevent staff from being open about their mistakes and learning from them. All these factors contribute to the UK having poorer outcomes on some measures than our peers in Europe, which is unacceptable.
>
> (2016, p. 3)

In 2014, the WHO strongly criticized the disrespectful and abusive treatment that women suffer while giving birth in hospital. In August 2019, Dubravka Šimonović, United Nations Special Rapporteur on violence against women, submitted a report entitled, "A human rights-based approach to mistreatment and violence against women in reproductive health services with a focus on childbirth and obstetric violence" to the UN General Assembly. In October 2019, a motion by the Parliamentary Assembly of the Council of Europe called on all member states, including the United Kingdom, to address obstetric and gynecological violence, which the motion asserts is a reflection of a patriarchal culture that is still dominant in society, including in the medical field. The motion declares that obstetric and gynecological violence is a form of gender violence that has long been hidden and is still too often ignored. In the privacy of a medical consultation or childbirth, women are victims of practices that are violent or that can be perceived as such. These include inappropriate or non-consensual acts, such as episiotomies and vaginal palpation conducted without consent or painful interventions without anesthetic as well as sexist behavior in the course of medical consultations, which has also been reported (Parliamentary Assembly of the Council of Europe, 2019).

Reflections

Historically, women have continued bearing children until the end of their reproductive age. What is different nowadays is that there is an increase in the age at which women give birth to their first child. The global fertility rate has fallen rapidly due to several major reasons: the empowerment of women, their growing access to education and increasing labor market participation, their opportunities for family planning, technological, sociocultural, and economic changes, as well as a rising cost of bringing up children, to which the decline of child labor contributed. We also need to take into account the impact of ART and the fact that women live longer as part of the changing field of motherhood. The fact is that women are having their first baby later in life and social and media debates tend to be played out through a discussion of the clinical problems about older women's ability to carry a pregnancy in their late thirties and forties and give birth to a healthy child. This tends to simplify and distort the science around fertility. Research by the British Pregnancy Advisory Service (BPAS, 2015) shows there is disproportionate concern among women about their fertility, and a tendency to overestimate the difficulties that may be encountered conceiving at the age of 35 or older.

The prevalent paradigm of medicalization in the institutionalized care of childbirth sees the woman who gives birth as an object of intervention and not as a subject of law, removing or detracting from their active role during the experience of pregnancy, childbirth, and the puerperium. Obstetric knowledge obtains greater legitimacy using a discourse aimed at showing medical intervention as the most effective way of decreasing maternal and infant mortality during childbirth. The institutionalization of the reproductive processes supplants the leading role of women in their own pregnancy, birth, and puerperium with the authority occupied by professional knowledge, thus bringing to fruition the asymmetry between obstetric professionals and patient. Foucault coined the term "medical gaze" to denote the dehumanizing medical separation of the patient's body from the patient's person (Foucault, 1963). Furthermore, the dehumanization of the delivery entails the naturalization of violence. The practices and instrumentation of obstetric treatment are exerted on women who are conceived merely as objects or bodies subject to intervention, and denied, implicitly, their human nature and their rights inherent to such.

All the participants in this study belong to the national racialized majorities of their respective countries, have university education, are economically independent, and have read and researched profusely about their assisted reproduction treatment and the type of delivery they wanted. All of them felt empowered by the use of ART and think it contributed to granting them more control over their body, reproduction, and motherhood. The majority were free of pre-existing medical conditions, led healthy lifestyles, and had no problems during their gestation. Nevertheless, none of those advantages protected them as laboring women at the hands of health professionals in public hospitals. Davis (2019) talks about obstetric racism which best describes Black women's reproductive care in the United States.

The obstetric teams in this study, according to the women interviewed, did not follow the recommendations of the WHO that women with an uncomplicated pregnancy at gestational age less than 41 weeks should not have an induction. If health professionals consider induction of labor to be necessary, they should discuss this option with women in advance, so that they understand the benefits and possible risks. In addition, if it is to be performed, women should be accompanied by health professionals at all times. Furthermore, the health professionals involved did not take into account the fact that none of the participants wanted a cesarean section.

The medical world is not exempt from the ageist and sexist attitudes prevalent in our patriarchal societies, for example, to be labelled "high risk" because the pregnant woman is over 35 years old, the constant warnings of the potential risks associated with pregnancy after 35 years; the tendency to perform a cesarean section on women over 35 years, despite having an uneventful pregnancy and being healthy. Moreover, ageism might aggravate the negative impact of other forms of discrimination, including sexism. Women who choose to become mothers on their own with the help of ART in their late thirties and onwards have decided to take control of their reproduction and choose when they want to become mothers. These women's life choices intensify moral judgements socially, in the media, and in the field of reproductive health, penalizing them for not complying with the norm of the heterosexual nuclear family, or procreating after the age of 35 years, or demanding their right to be informed regarding medical interventions on their bodies as well as their right to be treated humanely, with dignity and respect by health professionals.

Above all, these women wanted a successful birth. Thus, they submitted themselves to what obstetric specialists told them, having no other option. They had no room for maneuver other than accepting what was imposed or recommended. These women were not complicit in the appropriation that obstetric professionals made of their bodies. They were resigned to accepting medical decisions, trusting that at the end of it all they could hold a healthy baby. For the women in this study, the coveted "natural" birth proved a difficult goal to achieve.

References

American Society for Reproductive Medicine. (2012). *Age and fertility*. Retrieved from www.reproductivefacts.org/globalassets/rf/news-and-publications/bookletsfact-sheets/english-fact-sheets-and-info-booklets/Age_and_Fertility.pdf

Ayalon, L., & Tesch-Römer, C. (2017). Taking a closer look at ageism: Self- and other-directed ageist attitudes and discrimination [Editorial]. *European Journal of Ageing, 14*(1), 1–4. https://doi.org/10.1007/s10433-016-0409-9

Becker, G. (2000). *The elusive embryo*. Berkeley: University of California Press.

Boerma, T., Ronsmans, R., Aluisio, D y M., Barros, J. D., Barros, F. C., Juan, L., Moller, A. B., Say, L., Hosseinpoor, A. R., Yi, M., Rabello Neto, D., & Temmerman, M. (2018). Global epidemiology of use of and disparities in caesarean sections. Series Optimising caesarean section use. *The Lancet, 392*(10155), 1341–1348.

Bohren, M. A., Hofmeyr, G. J., Sakala, C., Fukuzawa, R. K., & Cuthbert, A. (2017). Continuous support for women during childbirth. *Cochrane Database of Systematic Reviews*. Retrieved from www.cochranelibrary.com/cdsr/doi/10.1002/14651858.CD003766.pub6/full

BPAS. (2015). *Becoming a mother: Understanding women's choices today*. British Pregnancy Advisory Service. www.bpas.org/media/y15hvqji/becoming-a-mother-understanding-womens-choices-today.pdf

Ciccarone, F., Tagliatesta, S., Caiafa, P., & Zampieri, M. (2018). DNA methylation dynamics in aging: How far are we from understanding the mechanisms? *Mechanisms of Ageing and Development, 174*, 3–17. https://doi.org/10.1016/j.mad.2017.12.002

Crawford, S., Boulet, S. L., Mneimneh, A. S., Perkins, K. M., Jamieson, D. J., Zhang, Y., & Kissin, D. M. (2016). Costs of achieving live birth from assisted reproductive technology: A comparison of sequential single and double embryo transfer approaches. *Fertility and Sterility, 105*(2), 444–450. https://doi.org/10.1016/j.fertnstert.2015.10.032

Davis, D.-A. (2019). Obstetric racism: The racial politics of pregnancy, labor, and birthing. *Medical Anthropology, 38*(7), 560–573.

Downe, S., Gyte, G., Dahlen, H., & Singata, M. (2013). Routine vaginal examinations for assessing progress of labor to improve outcomes for women and babies at term. *Cochrane Database of Systematic Reviews*. Retrieved from www.cochrane.org/CD010088/routine-vaginal-examinations-in-labor

Eijkemans, M. J. C., Poppel, F. v., Habbema, D. F., Smith, K. R., Lerido, H., & te Velde, E. R. t. (2014). Too old to have children? Lessons from natural fertility populations. *Human Reproduction*, 29(6), 1304–1312. https://doi.org/10.1093/humrep/deu056

Elmir, R., Schmied, V., Wilkes, L., & Jackson, D. (2010). Women's perceptions and experiences of a traumatic birth: A meta-ethnography. *Journal of Advanced Nursing, 66*(10), 2142–2153. https://doi.org/10.1111/j.1365-2648.2010.05391.x

European Perinatal Health Report. (2013). Health and care of pregnant women and babies in Europe in 2010. EURO-PERISTAT Project with SCPE and EUROCAT. Retrieved from www.europeristat.com/images/European%20Perinatal%20Health%20Report_2010.pdf

Foucault, M. (1963). *Naissance de la clinique: une archéologie du regard médical.* [The birth of the clinic: an archaeology of the medical gaze]. Paris: Presses Universitaires de France.

García-Lumbreras, S. (2019). What if I can't have children with my own ovules. Dexeus Clinic. Retrieved from www.dexeus.com/blog/en/latest/what-if-cant-have-children-with-my-own-ovules/

Goisis, A., Schneider D. C., & Myrskylä, M. (2017). The reversing association between advanced maternal age and child cognitive ability: Evidence from three UK birth cohorts. *International Journal of Epidemiology, 46*(3), 850–859. https://doi.org/10.1093/ije/dyw354

Gomes, M., Trocado, V., Carlos-Alves, M., Arteiro, D., & Pinheiro, P. (2018). Intrapartum synthetic oxytocin and breastfeeding: A retrospective cohort study. *Journal of Obstetrics and Gynaecology: The Journal of the Institute of Obstetrics and Gynaecology, 38*(6), 745–749. https://doi.org/10.1080/01443615.2017.1405924

Horsager-Boehrer, R. (2019). Why a scheduled C-section after 35 might be too risky. *Your Pregnancy Matters*. The University of Texas Southwestern Medical Center. https://utswmed.org/medblog/cesarean-over-35-risks/

Hospital Episodes Statistics (HES). (2018). Admitted patient care-provider level analysis. Retrieved from https://digital.nhs.uk/data-and-information/publications/statistical/nhs-maternity-statistics/2017-18

Huntriss, J., Balen, A. H., Sinclair, K. D., Brison, D. R., & Picton, H. M. (2018). Epigenetics and reproductive medicine. *BJOG. An International Journal of Obstetrics and Gynecology, 124*(13), 43–54. https://obgyn.onlinelibrary.wiley.com/doi/full/10.1111/1471-0528.15240

INE (Instituto Nacional de Estadística). (2015). Nacimientos por tipo de parto, tiempo de gestación y grupo de edad de la madre. [Births by type of delivery, gestation time and mother's age group]. Retrieved from www.ine.es/jaxi/Tabla.htm?path=/t20/e301/nacim/a2015/l0/&file=01011.px&L=0

Kitzinger, S. (2011). *Birth over 35*. London: Sheldon.

Korb, D., Goffinet, F., Seco, A., Chevret, S., Deneux-Tharaux, C., & EPIMOMS Study Group. (2019). Risk of severe maternal morbidity associated with cesarean delivery and the role of maternal age: A population-based propensity score analysis. *Canadian Medical Association Journal, 191*(13), 352–360. https://doi.org/10.1503/cmaj.181067

OECD. (2017). *Health Statistics: Health care utilisation*. Retrieved from https://data.oecd.org/healthcare/caesarean-sections.htm

O'Neill, C. (2015). The epigenetics of embryo development. *Animal Frontiers, 5*(1), 42–49. https://doi.org/10.2527/af.2015-0007

Parliamentary Assembly of the Council of Europe. (2019). Resolution 2603, Assembly debate on 3 October 2019. Document 14965, report of the Committee on Equality and Non-Discrimination, rapporteur: Ms Maryvonne Blondin. Text adopted by the Assembly on 3 October 2019 (34th Sitting). Retrieved from http://assembly.coe.int/nw/xml/XRef/Xref-DocDetails-EN.asp?fileid=28108&lang=2

Peter Singer, D. W. (1983). Symposium: 1. In vitro fertilisation: The major issues. *Journal of Medical Ethics, 9*, 192–195.

Petropanagos, A. (2015). Is advanced maternal age a public health issue? *American Journal of Bioethics, 15*(11), 56–58.

Präg, P., & Mills, M. C. (2017). Assisted reproductive technology in Europe: Usage and regulation in the context of cross-border reproductive care. In M. Kreyenfeld & D. Konietzka (Eds.), *Childlessness in Europe: Contexts, causes, and consequences* (pp. 289–309). New York: Springer Open.

Richards, S. E. (10 June, 2015). Women should never have an age limit on fertility treatment. *Time*. https://time.com/3914293/women-fertility-treatment-age/

Rothman, B. K. (2014). Pregnancy, birth and risk: An introduction. *Health, Risk & Society, 16*(1), 1–6. https://doi.org/10.1080/13698575.2013.876191

Schenker, J. G. (Ed.) (2011). *Ethical dilemmas in assisted reproductive technologies*. Berlin: De Gruyter.

Steiner, A. Z., & Paulson, R. J. (2007). Motherhood after age 50: An evaluation of parenting stress and physical functioning. *Fertility and Sterility, 87*(6), 1327–1332.

Tribunal de Justicia. (2006). Artículo 15. Ley orgánica sobre el derecho de la mujer a una vida libre de violencia. Venezuela [Organic law on the right of women to a life free of violence]. Retrieved from https://venezuela.unfpa.org/sites/default/files/pubdf/Ley_mujer%20%281%29_0.pdf

Warren, M. P., Shu, A. R., & Dominguez, J. E. (2015). Menopause and hormone replacement. In K. R. Feingold, B. Anawalt, M. R. Blackman (Eds.), *Endotext*. South Dartmouth: MDText.com, Inc.

WHO. (2018). *Recommendations: Induction of labour at or beyond term*. World Health Organization. https://iris.who.int/bitstream/handle/10665/277233/9789241550413-eng.pdf

5 The intersection of reproductive, work–life balance, early-education, and care policies

Introduction

The purpose of this chapter is to fill in the knowledge gap and our understanding of the complex interaction between women mothers-workers, sociocultural contexts, states, and social policies on reproduction, work–life balance, and early-childhood education and care. What barriers do women in the United Kingdom and Spain face on the road to becoming solo mothers by choice, and how do they navigate these challenges? Hence this chapter has the following aims: first, to identify the dominant approaches and the ways in which the normative assumptions and lack of reproductive, work–life balance, and early-education and care policies are challenged in the United Kingdom and Spain. Second, to examine the unequal access to assisted reproductive technology (ART) as a reproductive right to form a family. Third, to analyze the gendering of policies and the way responsibilities for caring needs are allocated between families and the state. Finally, it aims to explore how women juggle both earning a living and mothering their children, and how the welfare state and policy paradigms do not consider the unpaid care work, which contributes to gender inequalities in the labour market and other spheres of life. Drawing from this ethnographic study that focuses on Spain and the United Kingdom I will examine the effects of these policies, the social contexts in which they are applied, and the desires, frustrations, and needs expressed by the women interviewed. The data produced by this study reflects the different expectations the participants harbor in each country. I will argue that both in the United Kingdom and in Spain, women aged 35 and older who wish to have a child by themselves with the help of ART are discriminated against. In general, these women cannot access ART in their public health systems because they are considered "too old". Thus, those who decide to be solo mothers by choice have to plan years in advance, researching this option while saving money so as to be able both to pay for their ART treatment in private clinics and have a financial cushion to be able to afford early education and care for their children from 0 to 5 years old, particularly in the United Kingdom. These women then have to worry about whether they can balance their full-time job with motherhood. In some cases, they try to meet the expectations of their employers of working 70 h a week, while in others, they are forced to opt for part-time employment because their employers give no consideration to

DOI: 10.4324/9781003269755-6

work–life balance. Some are even pushed to the brink of becoming homeless. The chapter is divided into three sections. First, I describe the context of public policies in relation to work–family balance, and early education and childcare in the United Kingdom and Spain. Second, I examine the first obstacle that women encounter when they decide to start a family on their own using ART in the United Kingdom and Spain. Lastly, I analyze the interrelation of the second and third obstacles: how women juggle work and family life while managing the care and education of their children in both countries. .

Context

Within post-war Western Europe, the prevailing view of gender roles and responsibilities has been that of the woman as mother and primary caregiver, and the man as head of the household and principal breadwinner. These assumptions pervade all aspects of social and political behavior and sustain far-reaching political and socio-economic inequalities between men and women (Doepke & Zilibotti, 2019). In the context of policy-making, these assumptions give rise to "policy paradigms" based upon particular norms and values that help to define the policy problem as well as possible solutions. As Bacchi and Goodwin (2016) argue, policy problems do not exist "out there", but are socially constructed. Comparative analysis of childcare policy illustrates that childcare provision has typically been constructed as an educational policy issue and handled by policy-makers who have focused upon the educational needs of preschool-age children. In consequence, the employment needs of parents, and their needs regarding childcare, have rarely been considered (Randall, 2011). This is because many social rights of citizenship are dependent on participation in paid employment in the public sphere, whereas many women undertake unpaid care work in the household. Within the context of this policy paradigm, women are perceived primarily as mothers and dependents and, as such, are disadvantaged vis-a-vis men in terms of social rights, labour market position, and associated fiscal policies. Thus, the heterosexual nuclear family model has become the "great balancing mechanism" (Saraceno, 2008, p. 31).

As Randall (2011) argues, without affordable childcare, women's capacity to participate in the labour market and to be economically independent is severely constrained. The report by the European Commission/EACEA/Eurydice (2019) on early-childhood education and care confirms, notwithstanding the pressures for policy convergence within Europe, that significant national differences remain with regard to the amount, cost, and type of childcare provision available. This diversity confirms the continuing importance of state national welfare regimes and deeply embedded "policy paradigms" regarding the family, which have an important impact upon policies affecting women in the United Kingdom and in Spain. Work–life balance policies are intended to smooth out imbalances and conflicts between the contradictory demands of the labour market and family and personal care needs. These tensions become evident in decisions such as having a baby, when to have them, or where to live, and they affect aspects of our lives such as the care of our children and family members or our work careers. What we experience as individual problems and discomfort is embedded in deeper social and economic processes, which the design and application of public policies can help to shape, to one degree or another, according to their management and ambition.

To explore these questions, it is worth considering two related issues that dominate the popular discourse about motherhood and employment: (1) the difficulties of balancing motherhood and paid employment; and (2) the fact that mothers are having their first children later in life (Eurostat, 2020; UNICEF, 2011). Recent studies of gender discrimination suggest that in addition to inequalities in pay, women experience discrimination in terms of workload and the kinds of work available to them and in terms of the inflexibility of working hours (Social Issues Research Centre, 2012). According to the Global Gender Gap Report by the World Economic Forum (2016), it will take women 170 years to close the salary gap with men and to achieve equality in this area. A higher percentage of women are overqualified for their position, while the low number of women that reach management positions is worrying. According to Conde Ruiz and Marra de Artinano (2016, p. 21): "These glass ceilings are explained by the lack of work–family balance, the serious imbalance between qualification and job positions in the case of women, and gender stereotypes". Women suffer more from wage inequality and part-time work after the age of 35, when many of them choose to be mothers. This phenomenon is what experts call "the maternity penalty" (Correll et al., 2007) which carries with it a series of labour consequences for women: greater difficulty in finding employment, greater unwanted part-time work, and the request of practically all leaves of absence for reasons of family care, at 90.6% in Spain (INE, 2019).

Sara de la Rica, professor of economics, asserts that after the age of 30, when the decision is made to be a mother, women are forced to turn to occupations that are compatible with family responsibilities (de la Rica & Gorjón, 2016). Childcare and other caring tasks fall to women due to a lack of joint responsibility in the family unit and due to the shortfalls of public policies. Caring responsibilities are reasons for inactivity for almost 31% of inactive women, while this is only the case for 4.5% of men. The economic loss due to the gender employment gap amounts to around €370 billion per year for the European Union as a whole. "Taking action is both a social and an economic imperative. Improving gender equality could lead to an increase in GDP of up to €3.15 trillion by 2050" (European Institute for Gender Equality, 2021). In the case of the United Kingdom, in recent decades there has been a dramatic increase in the number of single-parent families. Thirty percent of households with children are headed by single parents, the large majority of whom are single mothers (Institute for Fiscal Studies, 2017).

The reason for the trend towards delayed motherhood in industrialized countries is multi-layered. However, a combination of interrelated factors is likely to be influential, such as access to contraception, increased duration in full-time education, and women's participation in the labour market (Broclchain & Beaujouan, 2012; Cory & Stirling, 2015). According to the OECD (2011), the United Kingdom spent 3.4% of GDP on family policies, Spain spent 1.2%, and the average in OECD countries was 1.9%. However, in terms of better outcomes for families, such as the ability to lift children out of poverty and gender equality, the United Kingdom lagged behind countries that spent less. Childcare costs in the United Kingdom are considerably higher than the 13% of overall family income it costs on average across the OECD. The United Nations Children's Fund (UNICEF) states that in relation to the composition of income-poor families with children, the proportion of sole-parent families varies from 24% in the United Kingdom to 7% in Spain (UNICEF, 2012).

First obstacle: solo motherhood in Spain and the United Kingdom and access to ART

The proliferation of ART has contributed to some of the major transformations in the Western kinship model over the past few decades. The use of biotechnologies has shifted the way reproduction is perceived and has impacted on contemporary family structures and dynamics. The new possibilities of reproduction, in vitro fertilization (IVF), gamete donation, and surrogacy have raised new opportunities for thinking about kinship that destabilize the nuclear heterosexual family framework. Even though heterosexual intercourse has ceased to be a necessary element for reproduction, it still operates as the global norm, from cultural customs, religious constraints to national laws. National laws mandate, for example, that in Europe the use of ART is allowed for heterosexual couples in every country, although many reserve it for married couples. Ten countries deny access to ART to solo women, up to 13 to lesbian couples, and surrogacy is banned in most countries in the world, and where it is allowed, strong restrictions against commercial surrogacy are in place (ESHRE, 2017). The extent of ART usage varies widely across countries, largely because of differences in the laws, the affordability and the norms surrounding child-bearing and conception. While restrictive national legislation can be easily circumvented by crossing national boundaries for ART treatments, questions of equity of access have been raised, as not all prospective parents can afford the treatment or to travel for it (ESHRE, 2018).

These restrictions are a source of a number of reproductive mobilities both from and to different European nations and other regions in the world, depending on the practice that is banned for different groups of people in the individual country. Actual numbers of solo individuals and same-sex couples using ART nationally or transnationally vary significantly across countries, there is not a reliable statistical picture. According to Salama et al. (2018), the major global markets for the cross-border reproductive care (CBRC) industry are as follows: (1) Belgium and Israel for IVF, (2) Denmark for sperm donation, (3) Spain and Czech Republic for egg and embryo donation, and (4) Russia and the United States for commercial surrogacy.

In 2006, it became legal for solo women and lesbian couples to access ART in Spain. Law 14/2006 on Human Assisted Human Reproduction in Spain (BOE, 2006) is one of the most advanced throughout Europe. Spain became a popular destination for international patients seeking ART treatments abroad. With the passing of the General Health Care Act in 1986, the right to healthcare was defined through a universal and decentralized national health system, which follows the model of a quasi-federalist state across Spain's 17 regions (López-Casasnovas, 2003). The Spanish law on gamete donations is different from that of other countries, protecting the anonymity of donors, which positively influences the high rate of egg and sperm donation, according to the experts. Although there are no accurate data on solo individuals or same-sex couples who use ART, medical practitioners indicate that the number is increasing.

For example, in 2012 in the Basque Country, Andalusia, or the Balearic Islands, a lesbian or a solo woman could access an assisted reproduction center on the national health system and undergo treatment to become a mother. However, in Madrid, Catalonia, Murcia, or Castilla-La Mancha this was not possible. In these regions women had no choice but to pay a private clinic to access ART. The law is the same for all, but their interpretation of the law may differ between the 17 regional health administrations, particularly the requirement that refers to the need for there to be "a diagnosis of sterility or a clinical indication". Furthermore, it depends on what the health departments understand by sterility: whether it is a strictly physiological question or if it goes further. If it is the latter, then it is not only about solving specific problems of reproductive disorders but also making motherhood accessible to different family models. Hence the accusations that the most restrictive positions in different regional health administrations are fueled by ideological arguments that limit the concept of family to the union formed by a man and a woman (Prats, 2012). Women may face waiting lists that take years to access treatment on the national health system, depending on the regional health administration. In the case of Andalusia, if women are older than 35 years, they have to pay for treatment privately. In the case of Madrid, the deadlines for receiving treatment counting from the first visit to the general practitioner in the six public hospitals that perform it vary from just over two to around four years (Medina & Mateo, 2019). On 5 November 2021, Spain's Health Minister in the socialist government signed an executive order reversing a ban on solo women and LGBTQ people from accessing free IVF services. The order restores the right of solo women and transgender people to receive IVF, one of the many forms of assisted reproductive health services covered under the country's public health system. This move comes nearly six years after the right-wing Popular Party government imposed a discriminatory policy in 2014 that restricted the treatments to heterosexual couples with fertility disorders (Borraz, 2021).

In the United Kingdom, according to the National Health Service (NHS, 2019), fertility treatment funded by the NHS varies across the United Kingdom, and waiting lists for treatment can be very long in some areas. The eligibility criteria can also vary. The coverage is based on infertility guidance from the National Institute for Health and Clinical Excellence (NICE, 2017). Nevertheless, individual NHS clinical commissioning groups (CCGs) make the final decision on who can have NHS-funded fertility treatment in their local area, and their criteria may be stricter than those recommended by NICE. This results in unequal access to treatment, as the final decision depends on local CCGs, which forces those potential mothers and parents who can afford it to go privately. As the price of private fertility treatment in the United Kingdom is high, some people go abroad for treatment where it is more affordable. Exact figures on just how much this group is growing are hard to find, as those who have treatment outside the formal clinic system in the United Kingdom are not captured in UK statistics. From 2005, the law was changed to allow children born through gamete donation to access identifying details of the donor. One of the consequences of this reform has been an acute shortage of donors (Turkmendag et al., 2008) and patients travelling to other destinations for treatment (ESHRE, 2017). Debbie, a 60-year-old Jewish white South African and British citizen who arrived in London in her twenties, gave birth when she was 43, with her own ovum and sperm from an anonymous Jewish donor. She is a head midwife at a public hospital in London (where I interviewed her), earning GBP 40,000 per year:

> I think the policies about help with getting pregnant are awful, because they're postcode luxuries, so it depends where you live, how much you get, what support you get. Who decides who is going to be a mother? Some pen pusher has decided in Brent, you can be a mother if you are under 28, and if you are married. In Greenwich I know a 32-year-old woman, and she's a lesbian and she got three IUIs (Intrauterine insemination – IUI – is a procedure that puts sperm directly inside the uterus, which helps healthy sperm get closer to the ovum). How do they decide this?

Estela, a 53-year-old university professor from Madrid, had her daughter when she was 44 years old through double anonymous ovum and sperm donation in a private clinic in the Spanish capital:

> I was told by my doctor that I could not receive treatment on the public health service. Only those women who were younger than 35 had access, and as there was a three-year waiting list, even those who were 32 years old when they applied for the treatment were not assured of getting it when they reached 35. It doesn't seem fair to me, since I've paid taxes my whole life. A smoker who's chosen to smoke all his life can receive treatment in public healthcare for any disease caused by his addiction. Why does he get it when I don't?

Professional legal advice warns that refusing treatment to patients based solely on sexual orientation, marital status, or women's age, may constitute illegal discrimination and does not have a sound ethical basis. Historically, women have continued to bear children until the end of their reproductive age. What is different nowadays is that there is an increase in the age at which women give birth to their first child (Eurostat, 2020). The decline in the global fertility rate can be attributed to various significant factors. These include the increasing access to education and participation in the labor market for women, the availability of family planning options, advancements in technology, changes in society and culture, and economic shifts. Additionally, the rising cost of raising children, along with the decrease in child labor, has also played a role in this decline. As part of the changing field of motherhood, we also need to take into account the impact of ART and the fact that women live longer. Women are having their first baby later in life, and social and media debates tend to be played out through a discussion of the clinical problems regarding older women's ability to carry a pregnancy in their late thirties and forties and give birth to a healthy child (BPAS, 2015).

All the study participants declared that they had a strong desire to be mothers. All had couple relationships in which they had wanted to share their wish to be mothers with their then partners, but were unable to do so, for many reasons. They therefore chose to pursue their dream of being mothers on their own, using ART. In all cases, participants state that it took them years to reach this decision, and that they prepared themselves mentally and financially to be able to cope with the costs that the decision entailed. An example of this is Joyce, 48 years old, who had her son 10 years ago with her own egg and a UK non-anonymous sperm donor from a private clinic. She is white British, a former consultant for a British multinational merchandise retailer earning GBP 100,000 per year. She talks about her journey to get the money to be treated privately and to have time off when she had her child to be able to care for and be with him.

> I had worked from the age of 21 until I was 38, when I had my son, that is, for 17 years. I worked before I was 21, in all the holidays between school and university and all of that as well, but full-time, seventeen years. Had a great career, earning bucket-loads of money. I didn't go on holiday for three years. I saved it all. I then took my three years off after my son was born.

A second example is Mila, a 38-year-old white French woman who has lived in London for the past 20 years, and works in human resources earning GBP 100,000 a year. She underwent ART in a private clinic in London and had a non-anonymous double donation (egg from a London donor and sperm from a donor abroad). She gave birth 8 months ago to her son: "It took me literally six years to get pregnant. So, during that time, I've saved a lot of money to pay for treatments, it also allowed me to take two years off to look after my son". Up until the time of their pregnancy, all the interviewees worked full time, and used their pay, savings, and family inheritance to invest their money in ART treatment. Emerald, who is white British from London, 65 years old with a 23-year-old son who was conceived through sperm donation and her own egg, used the IUI method for 30 cycles over three years. Isabelle, a white French resident in London, had seven IVFs over a five-year period.

However, one of the most obvious and long-standing ethical challenges surrounding assisted reproduction is the inequitable access to treatments and whether high costs interfere with procreative rights that include access to ART. Some argue that access to publicly funded ART is justified by the social advantages resulting from facilitating reproductive choice. A related argument is that state funding of ART fulfils the state's obligation to promote good health, including reproductive health (Zucker, 2014). Another more practical argument is that the public funding of ART will help halt the declining fertility rates and promote the addition of productive members of society. This may be an increasingly acceptable justification for the public funding of ART in countries experiencing a negative or flat population growth rate and seeking to develop public policies to alleviate the financial dilemmas of an aging population (Hoorens et al., 2007). Spain and the United Kingdom have very low fertility rates, 1.3 and 1.7, respectively, which may jeopardize the future of their welfare systems (The World Bank, 2019).

The interviewees perceive ART as a valuable instrument in attaining women's empowerment and autonomy by providing them control over their reproductive choices (Zucker, 1999). From a socio-legal perspective, the use of ART may, for many reasons, become an opportunity for women, providing they have the means, to re-appropriate their bodies in order to access maternity on their own or with a partner. The European Society of Human Reproduction and Embryology (ESHRE) has publicly opposed the introduction of restrictive ART legislation. All treatments known to be safe and effective should be available to all patients, who should be given the opportunity to make informed reproductive choices on the basis of sound scientific evidence.

However, the constant reference to "infertility" by the World Health Organization relies on heterosexual sex as a reference point, excluding "solo" patients and same-sex couples who currently seek fertility treatment. The sociologists Fledderjohann and Barnes (2018) have pointed out that statistics about infertility, which tend to be based on the reports of heterosexual couples, ignore the solo, less affluent, or non-heterosexual people who cannot have children for reasons that are only sometimes related to their bodies. On the surface, the effort to expand access to "infertility" treatment depends on the idea of equal rights. The World Medical Association's (WMA) Statement on ART, adopted by its General Assembly in October 2006, observes that "inability to become a parent without medical intervention (…) is a cause of major psychological illness and its treatment is clearly medical" (WMA, 2006). ART treatment is undoubtedly justified as a medical service and medical attention assisting the achievement of the goal of reproductive health. Its prohibition or undue obstruction is a human rights violation (Shencker, 2011).

The specific form taken by legislation with respect to the limits of reproductive technologies and the ways they are used can be interpreted as a reflection of the cultural conception of what motherhood is and should be, as well as of the social perception of fatherhood. Some feminist bioethicists argue that because women carry greater burdens with regard to biological and social reproduction, bioethical issues surrounding medically assisted reproduction are essentially debates over women's rights to bodily integrity and reproductive autonomy (Scully et al., 2010). Other bioethicists argue that issues surrounding procreation involve human rights (Donchin, 2004), regardless of gender, because the desire to have children and to participate in family life is a fundamental biological and social aspect of being human. Reproductive freedom or procreative liberty is essentially the individual right to have or avoid having children and to have the information and means to do so. Nevertheless, all the participants were denied access to ART on their national health services due to their age. If these women had not had the money to pay for their assisted reproduction treatment, they would not have been able to become mothers. Additionally, once they had confronted this first obstacle, a second and a third lay in wait: balancing the raising of a child with paid employment.

Second and third obstacles intertwined: work–life balance policies and early-education and care policies in the United Kingdom

Work–life balance policies are diverse due to the varying combination of public policy instruments that mobilize them, but also because of the cultural and institutional contexts that model them and are at the same time modelled by them. These contexts are known as "welfare–state regimes". More accurately, welfare regimes refer to qualitatively different arrangements between state, market, and the family in welfare provision. Although there are different typologies, the most used is that formulated by Esping-Andersen (1990), which distinguishes three ideal types of welfare–state regimes: the liberal or Anglo-Saxon, the conservative or Continental, and the social-democratic or Nordic regime. In European welfare studies, this classification is usually complemented by a fourth type, the Mediterranean welfare regime, which includes the southern European countries (Ferrera, 1996). Each of these regimes is characterized by a certain interaction between the public sector, the market and families, by fomenting a certain type of social stratification, by a different conception of citizens' social rights, and by a different significance of the meaning of the sexual division of labor and of gender relations. The so-called Anglo-Saxon regimes, such as the United Kingdom and Ireland, were historically characterized by an institutionalized individualist liberalism and familialism that have acted against universalist welfare policies. The private market and women have been the chief welfare providers with state social assistance reserved for those in marked poverty (Esping-Andersen, 1990). In other words, the welfare of families in these countries has essentially depended upon participation in the market, purchasing power and family connections and inheritance. Female employment rates are relatively high in these countries, although the relation of women with employment has traditionally been characterized by discontinuity and high rates of part-time employment.

In the United Kingdom between April and June 2019, three in four mothers with dependent children (75.1%) were in work, although only 44% of women were in full-time employment. This compared with 92.6% of fathers with dependent children who were in full-time employment. Almost 3 in 10 mothers (28.5%) with a child aged 14 years and under said they had reduced their working hours because of childcare reasons. This compared with 1 in 20 fathers (4.8%) (Vizard, 2019). In addition, a survey, conducted by Eurostat and published by the Office for National Statistics (UK), questioned more than 13,000 people in Britain, concluding that:

> Mothers may be more likely than fathers to throw a sickie at work when their children are ill and off school, and mothers of young children are also likely to stay at home to care for young children sent home from a nursery or by a childminder because they are ill.
>
> (Eurostat, 2019)

In the face of low state coverage, this labor pattern has become the prime balancing strategy of women and families. Hence, the Anglo-Saxon balance model has been called the "one-and-a-half breadwinner" model (Lewis, 2001). Families – meaning, in most cases, women – have to turn to private care services or to the help of other family members. However, only middle- and high-income families can afford the price of quality private care services, which creates a dual family stratification. The care service sector has traditionally been weak.

Preschool education and care policies: the United Kingdom

Early-childhood education and care (ECEC) refers to the care provision and education of children below primary school age outside of their family and home setting. The use of external childcare services is based on the combination of two factors: parental choice and the availability of such services. Childcare provision is central to many policies – child welfare, education, social, and even employment policies – and includes a wide typology of services: early-childhood care and education, emergency childcare, drop-in part-time babysitting services, care services for sick children, multi-purpose childcare facilities, out-of-hours childcare, or out-of-school care. This is not only essential for the healthy development of the child, but also to allow parents, especially women, to sustain or find employment. It is also a social inclusion measure that reduces the risk of poverty and social exclusion. The United Kingdom has a high overall education expenditure, but this includes the largest percentage of private expenditure of any European country. While similar levels are spent on education overall in the United Kingdom and Sweden, 20% of the total is private expenditure in the United Kingdom compared with 3% in Sweden. In the EUROSTAT "child wellbeing index", the Netherlands scores best, while the United Kingdom receives the lowest rankings. Fairly similar rankings emerge from the OECD Doing Better for Children (OECD, 2009), with the Nordic countries showing excellent results for child well-being, and the United Kingdom performing weakly. The average childcare costs for families with two children, in OECD countries, amounted to 13% of overall family net income. However, there are wide variations, ranging from 4% in Belgium to 33% in the United Kingdom. Payments for the cost of services for a two-year-old are lowest in Spain and highest in the United Kingdom (OECD, 2009, p. 68). All EU countries have some period of leave for parents of young children: half the countries (14) offer 6 months or less, with the United Kingdom having the shortest period at 6 weeks, while Spain offers 16 full-paid weeks.

Admission to formal compulsory schooling occurs at age of five in England. There is no consideration of a full-time entitlement to early-childhood services for all children under compulsory school age. Most forms of care are provided by the private sector. Another common form of childcare is that provided by friends, neighbors, and family members. From her research on forms of ECEC provision, Lloyd (2015) stated that the United Kingdom's early-childhood education and care system remains deficient in accessibility, affordability, and quality. Young children's rights and interests appeared to have been subjugated to the perceived interest of the economy and the government's deficit-reduction. According to Lloyd (2015), the absence of any consideration given to children's rights to quality early-years provision and of early childhood as a legitimate phase of life, more than as preparation for later educational outcomes, raises serious concerns about the future direction of early-years policy-making under the Conservative Government. In keeping with this, one participant in this study, Ellen, calls for public policies of work–life balance and of early-childhood education. She is 35 years old, from Dublin but living in London for the past ten years. She was treated in a private clinic and gave birth, in a London public hospital nine months ago, to a boy, the result of her ovum and a UK sperm donor. She works in patient safety management in the NHS and has a salary of GBP 63,000 per year.

> I think there should be significantly more support for childcare placements, and particularly for women in Britain. Governments make a big deal about equal pay, and wanting to support women in the workplace, and everyone knows that the biggest reason is around women going on maternity leave, and then childcare. If it was childcare vouchers, or support that is a tax relief on getting your child in, that just feels much more equal and fair. I also think there is social judgement: "You decided to have a child on your own, and now you can't do it, then you shouldn't have decided to do it". Children's centers should be free. I am paying for them with my taxes too … you'd avoid any sort of judgement because you've not been given it, you've just being allowed to access childcare the same way that everyone else is, so that you can get back to work, and earn money, and pay taxes.

At the national level, there is a need to develop a coordinated approach to address the issue of affordability, so that family income does not determine which children may benefit from quality early-childhood services. The limited access to services for preschool children, the variability in service provision across boroughs and regions, and the inequities in access to appropriate services for children in need of special support should be addressed. Ellen perceives that there are widespread negative attitudes towards solo mothers in the media and among the public, which can only further erode solo mothers' confidence and make them less likely to seek help. There is perhaps a role for government in challenging these negative perceptions, to help tackle the stigma of solo motherhood, and improve the well-being of solo mothers and their children. Boris Johnson, the former British prime minister, was strongly criticized on a radio show on 29 November 2019, for an article he wrote in 1995 in the *Spectator* stating that the children of single mothers were "ill-raised, ignorant, aggressive and illegitimate" children. In that radio show he refused to apologize. The journalist asked the prime minister, who has seven children, two from extra-marital affairs, how many children he had fathered, but he refused to discuss his own family. A caller explained that her children "suffered the stigma", demanding to know, "Why are you (Boris Johnson) happy to criticise people like me when you refuse to discuss your family?" (Merrick, 2019). Debbie and Grace explain, from their experiences, the lack of work–life balance policies and the sociocultural expectations that women be the family caregivers. Debbie, whom I mentioned earlier – a 60-year-old Jewish white South African and British citizen and a head midwife at a public hospital in London, earning GBP 40,000 per year – described how she experienced having a full-time job and being a full-time mother:

> I was awake every two hours, because the baby's screaming his head off and you've got to go to work the next day, and there's no-one else to take that baby. There are days when I crawled in here (the hospital), thinking "I don't know how I'm going to get through the day, and I've got to go and deliver babies and be safe?" I think childcare is a major issue in the UK. I got admitted to the hospital nursery, but it was still 8:00 a.m. till 6:00 p.m., and I worked 8:00 a.m. to 8:00 p.m. It didn't reflect any midwife's working hours. Childcare is so expensive! I used to pay £1000 per week to have a nanny between 8 a.m. to 7 p.m. Childcare in this country is so badly recognized and organized and so unsafe.

Cory and Stirling (2015) and Harknett et al. (2020) suggest that work and family policies need to adapt in order to keep up with these changing family structures, and ensure that all families are supported to balance work and care, by closing the gender pay gap, improving flexible working arrangements better to enable parents to respond to their family's needs, and by ensuring greater availability of affordable and high-quality childcare. Grace, a 51-year-old white British IT analyst who had her son 13 years ago with her own egg and non-anonymous sperm donor at a private clinic in the United Kingdom, explains the denigration that she perceives women, motherhood, and caregiving receive:

> I've never understood the degree to which motherhood seems to be denigrated to second best. Investing in the people of the future. I watch here in two central boroughs of London for 30 years, working in the community, and I look at the services for mothers and children and the amount of money that keeps disappearing. How much money has been wasted on Brexit to the detriment of everything else! How can you go out and get a job and get some self-worth if you can't afford childcare? Safe childcare, not leaving kids with your neighbors or playing downstairs. All I asked for my child was safe, affordable childcare.

Participants in this study have described the ways that they became invisible, that is, they perceived they lost their identity as a person of value the minute they left paid work or negotiated becoming part-time workers to take care of their children. It is this devaluing of and discrimination against caregiving that provides the common thread linking the experiences of women at the top and at the bottom. Claire is white British, 42 years old. She gave birth in a public hospital 19 months ago to her daughter who was conceived with her own egg and a sperm donor from the United States at a private London clinic. She explains the difficulty of balancing her job and her family life. She works as a senior manager at an American IT company that has 20,000 workers:

> I worried about can I afford to do this generally and will I cope with having a child 24/7 never being able to give it to anybody else? It was the whole how can I manage it all? Because I have a senior job, it's in an industry which generally requires long hours and commitment to your work. I need to earn a certain amount of money, particularly in London, to sustain a lifestyle to pay a mortgage, to pay for childcare. Then the pressures of being a solo parent where you have to do the pickup and the drop off and what that means to your working hours and your perceived commitment to the job. How am I going to do a job which involves 70 h a week?

Claire reveals her constant worry about her work, the hours they demand she invest, travel, and be absent from her home for days. However, she has a baby she breastfeeds and whom she cannot leave with a childminder all day long, but she is fortunate in having a sister who lives nearby and who can take care of her baby when the childminder's day ends. She mentions the male environment of her company, where most of the men are fathers, but whose wives are the ones who take care of the children, schooling, feeding and caregiving, or the management of it all, generally employing other women to take charge of these tasks. In fact, she does not know if she is going to be made redundant because she had informed her employers that she could not do all the tasks required of her:

> I'd be asked to go to Paris four days a week for the next four months, and I can't do that. The company I work for, it's run by white middle-class American men, it has huge challenges with diversity and inclusion. There's very few women, around 22%, the gender pay gap is terrible. They're not really geared up to women with families and flexible working. Whereas in a smaller organization they don't have the resources to focus on decent policies for working families.

Thus, her life has changed. She cannot go off anywhere just like that, she cannot work at weekends without having to calculate who will look after her daughter, how many hours, whether the childminder is available or not, if she has family members or a social network that can take care of her child, whether she can trust the person who does so, whether the baby will be happy with that person. There are many decisions and worries that need to be dealt with before accepting the task that her company sets her or not. It is clear which set of choices are more valued today. Workers who put their careers first are typically rewarded; workers who choose their families are overlooked, and overworked. Ellen, mentioned earlier, faces similar problems:

> I've extended my maternity leave. I'm going back part time and using annual leave. My mum will hopefully come over from Dublin once a month to do the extra days because the nursery is so expensive, I can't really afford it. I get no support because they've changed the rules and it disproportionately affects single parents. It used to be household income, and now it's individual income,

> so a couple could both be earning £49,999 each, so they earn almost £100,000, and have two people, so they can share childcare, they would still qualify for child benefit. I'm one person, but because I earn more than £50,000, I don't get anything.

Her mother has to help her, flying in from Ireland, and she makes clear the discrimination faced by solo parents, mostly mothers, from the measures of the British government. According to Garnham (2018), the chief executive of Child Poverty Action Group, when the bill introducing Universal Credit (UC) was published in 2011, it was criticized on how the policy was flawed. Women are disadvantaged in UC in a number of ways. First, it resembles a return to the 1950s family wage model. Second, it entrenches traditional divisions of labor. The insistence of UC on dividing a couple with children into a "main earner" and a "main carer" (or second earner) is problematic. Third, the benefit cap disproportionately affects women: of households subject to the benefit cap, 93% have children, 72% are lone parents (76% with children under five and 31% with a child under two). The vast majority of these will be women. These claimants have young children so they face barriers to work, and cannot find affordable housing. Those with babies and toddlers are not required to look for work in the benefits system, yet they are still hit by the cap. Solo parents, mostly mothers, are twice as likely to receive less money than to gain financially when moving from the old benefits system to UC, according to new research which criticizes the "harsh treatment" of the claimants (Talbot, 2021). Katya is a case in point. She is 47, a Russian Jew who lived in Israel before migrating to London twenty years ago. She holds a Master's degree and works as a mental health nurse at an NHS hospital, being considered a key worker. It took her 3 years to take the decision to become a solo mother with the help of ART. Then she travelled to a private clinic in Spain and got an embryo adoption from a double anonymous donation. She had the embryo implanted and flew back to London on the same day. She had given birth just five weeks earlier when I went to her shared flat for the interview. Her baby was asleep and she was very distressed. She told me that the council wanted to evict her from the two-bedroom flat that she shared with another tenant. They wanted to remove her on the premise that, because she had had a baby, she was no longer just one person. According to the council, she and her baby "were overcrowding the flat". Her eyes filled with tears: she only earned GBP 30,000 a year and the rent for a small flat near the hospital where she worked would cost her GBP 1,300 a month. She could not afford it: it would consume three-quarters of her salary. Despite this situation, the council was pressuring her with threatening letters. They had shown her social housing where there were too many people, many with problems of addiction or mental illness. She did not feel "safe" with her baby in this type of housing. She said: "the council does not care about single mothers". During the first hour of the interview, her account was constantly interspersed with "it's my choice": "I chose to have a baby". According to her, the state should not be made responsible for her and her baby: "you make your bed you lie in it", she would repeat. She did not criticize the council for: (a) wanting to remove her from the flat with her five-weeks-old baby; (b) not providing affordable housing for key workers; or (c) not paying key workers enough money, thus forcing her to live through this pitiful situation. Nevertheless, in the second hour of the interview, Katya asserted that there should be affordable housing, quality education, and care for children aged 0–5 available to everyone.

Sandher (2019) describes the United Kingdom's key workers as foreign-born, working dangerously, and earning less: "More than one in five Health and Social Care workers were born abroad and they have seen their hourly earnings fall by 7.5% since 2010". The OECD (2020) stated that in COVID-19 pandemic, we are all relying on immigrants who are over-represented in key worker categories. Stringent conditions for receiving welfare benefits are increasingly common in high-income countries. Katikireddi et al. (2018) argue that requiring lone parents with school-age children to seek work as a condition of receiving welfare benefits adversely affects their mental health. Research already shows low-paid female workers are five times more likely to experience depression. Pickavance (2020) argues that now is the time to "reset" our cultures by placing worker well-being center stage, and to think about employment practices and rates of pay that make saving more likely. Childcare must become an urgent strategic imperative. Another example is Susan, 54, a white British Londoner, who works as a freelance criminal solicitor. She is the mother to a 10-year-old boy who was conceived with the help of a double anonymous donation (egg and sperm) at a private clinic in Spain, and gave birth at a public hospital in London. She speaks about her efforts to balance family and work:

> I do legal-aid criminal work and there's no money, terrible hours and no flexibility. This is the problem with the job I got in the summer, they said to me: "We want you to work in the city", and I was like, "Okay, that's fine", "You've got to be there at nine o'clock", I said, "I can't be there at nine o'clock because I've got a child that I had to drop at school at 8:55, I can be there at 9:30 and I can do a half an hour lunch, if you want me to". Not even prepared to discuss it! Why do I have to physically be there? I've got a mobile phone, if you need to speak to me, you just call me. The reality is I'll probably be at court, so why do you need me to physically be in the office? Very, very old-fashioned ways of seeing things.

When law firms and corporations hemorrhage talented women who reject lockstep career paths and question promotion systems that elevate quantity of hours worked over the quality of work itself, the problem is not with the women (Slaughter, 2015, p. 15). Plenty of women are juggling paid work and childcare but still they run up against obstacles created by the combination of life circumstances and the rigid inflexibilities of their workplaces and the lack of public infrastructure of care. The workplace is discriminating in favor of workers who can outsource caregiving to someone else. Governments and employers assume that care work is not work that really matters, even though it is essential to the very brain formation and growth of the young. Care work is work. It is not self-indulgent; it is radical and necessary (Federici, 2012; Ahmed, 2014). Systematically marginalizing care "furthers the myth that our successes are achieved as autonomous individuals and, as such, we have no responsibility to share the fruits of our success with others" (Lawson, 2007, p. 5).

Susan does not opt out of her job, she is shut out by the refusal of her bosses to make it possible for her to fit her family life and her work life together. These women need reliable work at a decent wage that allows them the following: to save for a rainy day; access to affordable, high-quality day-care and early-education programs; paid days off and family leave for the inevitable times that their children or other loved ones who depend on them are sick or in need; and recognition and respect for the care they do (Slaughter, 2015, p. 24). Yet today the United Kingdom does not provide affordable day-care, early-education, and afterschool programs that take up the caregiving slack. They do not provide sufficient paid leave that any worker can use when a child is sick. The result is that the mother with dependent children must patch together an unstable and unreliable network of caregivers in ways that sharply hinder her ability to succeed at her job. For working-class and middle-class women, the struggle to balance caregiving and breadwinning is a daily grind and often the tipping point that may drive them into poverty. When I asked Susan: "Why do you think there is no change in policies?" she replied:

> I don't think this government is particularly interested. They say they want parents to go back to work but it seems to be more of a stick than a carrot, most of the time. So, "We'll take your benefits away, unless you work". I think mostly women make it work and they're the ones who are going home. It is not only a matter of gender. The way it's organized, the people who run the business make the money and the people who do the job get paid very little. So, I have encountered women who have got nannies like a Queen's Counsel, who are partners and say: "Well, I can manage it, why can't you?" Yes, even though they're paying their staff £35,000 per year and they're probably earning £90,000, and they've got husbands who are earning if not the same then certainly enough to pay for a nanny. So, of course she can make it work and when I raised it, she said, "Well, you can't do this job unless you work full-time", and that was basically her view. So, even the women who are running it don't see it. The fact that the majority of people who are in Parliament have come from such a privileged background. It goes back to Norman Tebbit "getting on your bike". It's not actually having any real sense of how people who are not them are living. The other thing I find very hard, because I've been to lots of these meetings is that I'm sitting in a room full of men most of the time. The only other woman might be the person taking the notes. I can sit there and tell them all my ideas for hours but they've got no vested interest in there.

In 1981, at a time when the British Conservative Government of Margaret Thatcher was being blamed for high unemployment, a member of her cabinet, Norman Tebbit, gave a speech to the Conservative Party Conference and said: "I grew up in the '30s with an unemployed father. He didn't riot; he got on his bike and looked for work and he kept looking till he found it" (Daily Telegraph, 1981).

The implication being that he thought people who were long-term unemployed were simply too lazy to find jobs. The Queen's Counsel is not accommodating of work–family conflicts, she has absorbed the values and practices of the system where she has succeeded, and perpetuates it in demanding that others make it the same way, discounting social class, ethnicity, and solo motherhood as factors that obstruct equality. Only 34% of all members of parliament (MP) are women, only 10% of all MPs are from minority ethnic backgrounds (Audickas & Cracknell, 2020). Increasing the supply of affordable, good-quality childcare would help solo parents, the majority mothers, to move into work. The literature has demonstrated the importance of arranging childcare as a key element of lone-parent employability services, and the impact of affordable and readily-available childcare can be seen in international comparisons (Graham & McQuaid, 2014).

In the case of the participants living in London they, in general, have interiorized the discourses of successive governments and part of the media that grumble about a "nanny state" (a term of British origin that conveys a view that a government or its policies are overprotective or interfering unduly with personal choice. The term "nanny state" likens government to the role that a nanny has in child rearing). Thus, most of the London participants follow the principle of "you made your bed, now lie in it" – I've chosen to be a solo mother by choice, so I'll take on paying for the ART because I'm around 35 or older, I'll take on paying for the education and care of my child until the age of five because there are no state policies of education and care for this age group, at the same time as needing to work for a salary that will pay the mortgage or the rent in the most expensive capital in Europe (Statista, 2021).

The London participants have, in general, also interiorized the discourses of British governments regardless of their educational level, all of them having had the benefit of a university education, some with masters and doctorates, and some have even transgressed the rules of their religious community and the opinions of their families against their having children on their own with the aid of ART, and have gone ahead with their decision. In that part of their lives, they were brave and transgressive with respect to their families of origin, their social networks, their religious community, or their milieu. However, in other parts of their lives, such as demanding from the state access to public assisted reproduction for women aged 35 years or older, work–life balance policies or fair education and care policies, they were not so outwardly brave. They have taken in the discourse that demonizes the "nanny state", one that blames solo mothers, the poor, or the unemployed who have no choice but to seek aid from the state, and socially stigmatizes them. They find it humiliating to need state support, something which for them goes hand in hand with the idea of personal failure.

The British author Owen Jones states that the more unequal the society, the greater the need to demonize in order to justify it. According to Jones, the case of the United Kingdom is key because, particularly since Thatcherism, the change occurred whereby poverty and inequality were no longer presented as social problems but as failures of the individual (Jones, 2015). Tebbit's phrase, "get on your bike", became a national cliché. The huge inequalities and the shift from the need for a collective response to governmental individualism are especially notable in the United Kingdom, where, in general, the media maintain and support this discourse.

This may explain how the London participants have internalized the public discourses on what is success and failure, and applying for state benefits is represented as begging from the state. Because these women have chosen something individually as a personal option – having a family outside of the heterosexual nuclear family norm – means that they have to pay a price that must come out of their own pocket: private ART treatment, the private clinic, the importation of semen, or travel to other countries to attain egg donors or double donation because in the United Kingdom this type of treatment may not be provided due to a lack of egg donors (Turkmendag et al., 2008), or psychological treatment to treat their bereavement for the many times that, despite the ART, they have not been able to get pregnant or have had miscarriages (García-Lumbreras, 2019).

They also have to pay the price for the fact that their employers (private or public, such as the NHS) have not established work–life balance measures. It is they who, preparing the way for years, have saved money or changed their place of residence to where they could have easier access to good preschools to care for and educate their children, or who have to work part-time and draw on their savings because their employers will not consider a balance between family and work. Lastly, the UK participants perceive that the successive governments view the raising and care of children as a private, individual matter, not a collective one: "look after yourselves", abandoning any co-responsibility of the state or employers with regard to work–life balance policies or of implementing public education and care policies for the preschool population.

This lack of public policies in the reproductive, labor, and education spheres translates into an obstacle course in which the women have to fend for themselves in order to be mothers and balance their motherhood with their career. Due to the pandemic, they have also become their children's teachers in a home-schooling context. Yet despite the worst conditions that the London participants suffered with regard to the lack of educational or care policies for their preschool children, despite the fact that only a minority of them could count on the sporadic help of their family and social networks, despite the fact that some of them were forced to become part-time workers, they did not, in general, demand access to public reproductive treatment, or work–life balance policies, or public policies of care and education for children aged 0–5 that would enable and guarantee that they and future generations might have and raise their children and work for a decent wage. They did not demand them, even though if women do not have the financial means, the option of being mothers on their own is impossible.

Second and third obstacles intertwined: work–life balance policies and early-education and care policies in Spain

Guillén and León (2011) argue that the countries of southern Europe – Portugal, Spain, Italy, and Greece – form a welfare model with a different tradition and characteristics. These countries share certain political and institutional peculiarities: precarious labor markets with high unemployment rates; income transfer programs characterized by high protection in certain cases (pensions) and large areas of exiguous protection or total lack of protection (dependence; housing); a strong private sector presence in many areas of service provision; a peculiar mix between public and private sector; and a familialism that does not only involve the nuclear family but also the extended family (Naldini, 2006). It is precisely family solidarity that has traditionally substituted for the lack of, or little flexibility in, public and private care services.

The relation of women with employment has been characterized – unlike what has taken place in Anglo-Saxon and Continental countries – by continuity and full-time work. However, Mediterranean familialism has been undergoing a spectacular transformation in recent years (León & Migliavacca, 2013; Calzada & Brooks, 2013). This is shown in the transformation of the attitudes towards the family and lifestyles, in the high employment rates of women between the ages of 25 and 49 years in Spain and Portugal – these rates are similar to Sweden and Denmark – and in the growing development of early-childhood education services and attention to dependence. Nonetheless, the feminization of part-time work is a reflection of the forced choice of this type of contract that women take in order to be able to care for their children or family members in a situation of dependence, or to take care of other family or personal responsibilities.

According to data from the Spanish National Institute for Statistics (INE, 2019), of the 18,535,900 households that were registered in the 2018 Ongoing Household Survey in Spain, 10.1% (1,878,500) are one-parent families. Of these, 81.9% (1,538,200) are headed by a woman. Irene, a 39-year-old Spanish architect from Madrid, who has lived in London for six years, has an eight-months-old baby conceived through anonymous sperm donation and was treated at a private clinic in Madrid. She works in a construction company in London with a salary of GBP 65,000 a year, but now she has to ask to become part-time to be able to look after her baby, as she complains that the crèches in London are very expensive. In our interview at her home in Madrid, she compares Madrid and London with regard to bringing up a child, work–life balance policies, and early-education and care policies.

When I went to the United Kingdom, I was surprised by how sexist it is, much more than Spain. A crèche costs 1,500 quid a month. What family can pay that? The woman stops working and in a few years has several children in a row and her professional career vanishes, her husband's flourishes. If you have two children under three, preschool rises to £3000 a month. In the end women give up their professional career. In Spain it is looked down upon if the state does nothing when someone needs help. There are many public crèches and you don't pay more than €190 a month. In the United Kingdom they are very individualist, there is a negative conscience about state protection of the individual, it is frowned upon to request help from the state. I've paid taxes all my life and I believe that the state should be there to provide education and care from the age of 0, that's why I pay taxes.

She expects and demands her rights to early-childhood education and care once maternity leave has ended. She wants and needs to continue working. This demand is heightened in the case of a solo-mother family, since it is not founded upon the premise of the hetero-patriarchal middle-class nuclear family in which the woman stays at home to look after the children and do the housework without any social or monetary recognition, or she must make a "forced choice": work part-time and work in the home caring for the children, thus reflecting the ideology of the male breadwinner and the female caregiver. Irene continues:

> I see English society as still very conservative, the men very chauvinist in many cases, paternalist and condescending. My project manager, a 60-plus-year-old man, calls me "cutie pie" at work. The fact that he calls me "cutie pie" already devalues me. You have to demonstrate a thousand times over your worth because you are a woman and a foreigner. For the mere fact of having an accent it seems that you are worth less as a person.

Irene debunks her idea of the United Kingdom as one of the most advanced countries and suffers in person the degrading treatment of her boss for being a woman and unequal treatment for being a foreigner with a particular accent. She also compares public early-childhood education in Spain with the necessarily private equivalent in the United Kingdom. Many children start in preschools straight after Spain's four-month statutory maternity leave. New mothers are entitled to 16 weeks fully paid leave, and as of 2021, fathers have the same right. Even though compulsory education does not begin until the age of six, the OECD reports that Spain has had nearly full enrolment in early-childhood education and care. In 2018, 98% of 3–5 year-olds were enrolled in early-childhood education and care programs in Spain, compared with 88% on average across OECD countries (OECD, 2021). Preschools run by the state usually provide childcare for the whole day and include lunch.

The costs are subsidized by the state and vary depending on income. For example, in Madrid, for the academic year 2020–2021, families whose per capita income is equal to or less than €5,644 a year pay a monthly school fee of €58, while families whose per capita income is higher than €25,725 a year pay €188 a month. There is a reasonable amount of flexibility in terms of hours of attendance and parents can choose mornings, afternoons, full days, or just a few days per week. State education is free of charge in Spain from preschool to 18 years of age, although in some regions parents may be asked to pay for books, other materials, and extra-curricular activities. In the case of the Spanish participants of this study who live in Spain, they all stressed the importance of their own families in the raising of their children, when their maternity leave ended and they could access public preschools. For example, in the case of Nerea, a sociologist who had her daughter with sperm donation at the age of 35 years, her mother offered to look after her daughter while Nerea worked:

> In order to make the decision to be a solo mother by choice, I counted on my mother, and she told me that she was retiring around that date, and that

she would help me for as long as needed. Having my mother's help was very important. Also having a public preschool where I took my daughter from when she was a baby.

Carol, a 47-year-old from Barcelona, had her daughter through double donation at a private clinic nine months ago. She is a self-employed IT designer, and her father said to her:

> We love you, we see that becoming a mother is very important to you and as you catch us in old age and we can't help you much, logistically speaking, we have decided to give you this money so that you can use it for the private clinic or for nannies or for whatever you need.

Her parents and siblings live nearby and if she needs to leave her baby for a while, her parents look after her. María, a 46-year-old from Seville who had her two children, now four and six years old, through sperm donation from different donors at a private clinic, is a civil servant and lives close to her mother and siblings. She underlines the importance of living close to a preschool that is connected to a primary school that charges very little.

> I'm the oldest and I have a sister and a brother who are married with children and they have had to help me daily. I also help them. I chose the school that was close to my mother's house and mine, because if I go to work and it's my mother who has to pick them up at a given time because they get sick, I wanted to make that task easy for her, as she's helping me.

However, employers do not make balancing work and family easy. Lia, aged 38, the daughter of Argentinian exiles, who lives in Madrid and is a lecturer at a public university, is the mother of a three-year-old boy, conceived through sperm donation at a private clinic, and a seven-year-old girl, from her last relationship. She complains of the unequal treatment by the law towards solo-mother families:

> In the case of solo mothers by choice, they should add the paternity leave to the maternity leave so as not to discriminate against the child in comparison to heterosexual nuclear families who can benefit from adding the maternity and paternity leaves together. I requested it in writing from my university. The law does not see it that way. Moreover, I gave classes until 9 p.m. with my six-month-old baby. I had to pay a childminder. Neither the Department, nor the university equality unit that the university boasts about, helped me in anything.

Elaborating on the topic of universities throughout my academic career in Spain and the United Kingdom there have been many occasions when I have been faced with sexism and discrimination . One such experience occurred at a public university in Spain, when I was pregnant, a senior male professor proposed that since I would give birth in the second semester, I should change my teaching to the first semester. This would never have been suggested to a male professor who was going to be a father. The second sexist episode occurred at the end of that same meeting, when another senior male colleague told me that my husband could take paternity leave so that I could dedicate myself more to my teaching, assuming that I had a (male) partner. That is, he offered a suggestion that I did not request, setting himself up as the expert on how to manage my maternity leave. A different episode occurred at a faculty board meeting with the dean, whom I asked if I could teach one of my subjects later in the morning in order to balance my work and family life (my daughter was then 8 months old and the nursery did not look after babies in the early mornings). The dean replied that all academic staff had raised their children and that they had managed without having to change schedules. What she did not mention was that in her home there were two salaries, hers as a tenured professor and her husband's, as a member of the regional government, with which they paid a woman to do the household chores and to take their children to and from school. The dean was not accommodating of work–family conflicts, she had absorbed the values and practices of the patriarchal system where she had succeeded, and perpetuated it. . Only 22.5% of women are full professors despite the fact that 49.8% of women are lecturers on temporary contracts in public universities in Spain (Ministerio de Universidades, 2020). Some years later at a public university in London where I worked as a researcher in a department dedicated to family studies, and whose "staff get-togethers" were scheduled in the afternoons, ignoring the fact that school hours ended at 3.30 p.m. and that I could not attend (nor other members of the department who were mono-parental families) unless I found a childminder and paid her GBP 12 an hour. However, after less than 8 months, my daughter had already been looked after by five different childminders, women for whom their studies and other jobs were more important than babysitting a few hours a week. One of them made my daughter accompany her into the bathroom of my home when she was menstruating to "teach" her what it meant to have periods. My daughter was 7 years old. I had assumed that the fact that this department focused on family studies, in particular, would mean that it would have work–family balance policies as one of its priorities. I wrote to the head of the department, a white British professor, about it; but I was wrong: she did not reply and nothing was done (Bravo-Moreno, 2022). According to the Higher Education Statistics Agency, United Kingdom, only 28% professors (defined as senior academic appointments which may carry the title of professor) were female in 2021, male professors continue to outnumber females by three to one. The percentage of female professors increased by one percentage point year on year from 2013–2014 until 2019–2020 and has remained at 28% for 2020–2021 (HESA, 2022).

Rosa is 54 years old from Madrid, is the founder of a solo-mothers-by-choice association, a journalist, and the mother of a 14-year-old adopted daughter and a 10-year-old girl conceived though sperm donation at a private clinic. She explains:

> We (solo mothers by choice) only have the resources of one adult person to maintain the household: half that of a two-parent family. One single source of income, a more limited support network, half the leave in terms of personal days, holidays, even due to birth, fostering/adoption, and breastfeeding. We also only have two hands and one mind to run the ship. Mental health is fundamental for maintaining and accompanying the little ones.

Thus, investment is needed in work–life balance, which is understood as social co-responsibility. The measures should address family diversity and be adapted to the needs of all types of families. Treating what is different equally creates inequality and discrimination, according to Lola, founder of the Federation of Single Mother Associations (FAMS):

> We already began the state of emergency of the pandemic at a disadvantage, which we have been making known to the administrations and social agents for some time now, because of a system that revolves around the traditional family and that penalizes us in different areas, both financially and in terms of balance. Through FAMS we have launched the campaign #ConciliarDificilEquilibrio (work–life: difficult balance) to show the juggling acts we have to perform, the difficulty of balancing all the factors: work, education, health, care, self-care, in a context without social co-responsibility from the public sphere, creating greater inequalities and gaps in our families. The fundamental role of caregiving in this society needs to be recognized and valued, in economic terms too. This crisis is making it all clear in all its rawness. Society needs a work–life balance plan in the short term with urgent measures so that the consequences do not fall on the shoulders of women and children harming families like our own who started the COVID-19 game several squares behind the starting square.

In 2021, the European Parliament passed two resolutions: one to apply gender perspective in the COVID-19 crisis, and the other with the EU strategy for gender equality (European Parliament, 2021). These are non binding resolutions that do not compel the European Commission to modify its proposals or the member states to apply particular measures. Instead, they fix priorities. One of these priorities is the creation of a European Pact for Caregiving, because the current Work–Life Balance Directive – that must be transposed into member states' national law by August 2022 – "proves insufficient". The parliament asks its member states for measures for "the promotion of men's equal role as carers, thereby tackling gender stereotypes in take-up of either paternity, maternity, or both, leave (Wayne et al., 2016) the recognition of the role of informal carers by ensuring their access to social security and their right to pension entitlements". There are mentions of single-parenthood in the main design mechanisms and strategies, planning, evaluation, and monitoring of public policies that address child and family protection. However, these policies have the two-parent family model as their starting point, despite recognizing the protective needs of solo-parent families due to their particular vulnerability. These references have not mobilized administrations to look for regulation at the state level that recognizes the condition of solo-parenthood as a family model; rather it has served as a reminder that another type of family exists when situations of particular vulnerability to poverty and risk of social exclusion occur. In short, social policies do not take this group specifically into account as a family model that should be protected as such; instead, intervention is structured as a form of relief through complements in benefits, tax relief, grants, and income guarantees.

All the Spanish participants living in Spain spoke of how to improve the lives of solo-mothers-by-choice families with political demands. In the interview I conducted with an ex-president of the "Single-mothers by Choice" association, she explained:

> One of the achievements of this association is reaching a greater number of women, letting them know that we exist and that they are not alone. Another is legal recognition. The administrations cannot make laws on something that is not recognized as such. If it does not exist, it does not have rights. For example, the children of two-parent families have, from the beginning of 2021, 32 weeks of leave (maternity and paternity), and our children only have 16. The approach is twofold: the right of women to choose their family model, and the right of the child to have the same rights as other children regardless of the filiation from their mother or father. This is not being met. Somehow they state that our children can have the same rights, but until now nobody has bothered to legislate on the matter. And we also want a solo-parent family law that would see us as just another family model. This includes families that are solo-parent due to the death of one parent, due to circumstance, due to divorce where the father does not take care of the children, and so on. A law that generations will benefit from. What we want is the raising of children in diversity with equal rights: making visible, forming a network, and protesting are our pillars.

One of the most well-known spheres in which violence is wielded against women is the economic. Whether in couple relationships, the labor market, or the division of housework and care work, women undergo a great deal of hardship. The economist Carmen Castro (2020) explains that the Istanbul Convention – the most important international treaty on the human rights of women – states that all these types of economic violence form a part of gender-based violence, alongside physical or psychological violence. As such, they are a serious assault on the human rights of women and girls. Castro adds: "Caregiving has to be part of that economic and social change and to do so through an agreement on a different distribution of times, divisions and incomes" (Castro, 2020, p. 58).

Conclusions

In this chapter, I have analyzed, first, how these women address the need to turn to the private provision of a fundamental human right: the creation of a family. One of the long-standing ethical challenges surrounding assisted reproduction is the unequal access to treatments and whether high costs hinder procreative rights that include access to ART. Second, I have examined how "solo" motherhood is a complex reality of social typology, in which different forces from different institutions, social agents, and powers converge, interact and affect the women in this sample and broader groups.

In neither of the two countries that I focused on is there a framework of integrated public policies and measures at state level that regulate and recognize solo-parenthood as part of family diversity on an equal playing field with other family models. The absence of a national law hinders there being any homogeneous legal, social, educational, economic, and labor treatment of the rights of solo-parent families. This fact does not mean that they can all be put in the same boat without differentiating between, and attending to, the needs of each of them. The inclusion of single parenthood in public policies and in social solutions requires the breaking of the monocular approach that identifies it with poverty. The aim is to provide an analysis capable of observing, capturing, and confronting how situations of discrimination affect women-mothers-workers by themselves – and their children.

This is done not only from a multidimensional gender perspective but also through the intersection of the inequalities faced by the members of these families due to economics, national origin, gender, functional capacities, education, culture, and so on. The solo-parent family is made completely invisible when it comes to designing public policies and establishing measures for equality and protection. Therefore, tackling this question requires taking on approaches that can reveal the multidimensionality of the problem in order to guide public policies and have a bearing on the quality of the lives of these families. Family and personal networks should not be the ones responsible for solving daily difficulties, and the state should not intervene only in a subsidiary fashion when all else fails.

The consequence of this legal framework and public policies is that they perpetuate both the two-parent family model and the barriers that prevent women from freely choosing what personal and affective life they wish to have. This system worsens female poverty and, in particular, the poverty of single-parent households, because it leaves them without protection. An effective policy of equality should address the needs of women who fulfil caregiving and breadwinning roles, as well as those who work as domestic workers, child-minders, and early-education teachers. Solo-mother families must not be an exception; they must be part of the norm, of the normality of family situations that public policies need to address. Only in this way can solo-motherhood cease to be associated with poverty and risk of exclusion and to articulate integrated policies. By recognizing solo-motherhood as part of family diversity, it will be shown: (a) that all forms of family have common needs related to supporting life (emotionally and materially); and (b) that certain family realities (e.g., solo-parent, immigrant, large, same sex, blended families, families at risk of or in a situation of exclusion) present particular needs that must be addressed attending to the needs of each of them.

Early education and work–life balance policies should be key tools for attaining a wider outlook, a truly co-responsible approach that engages and commits institutions and businesses, men, and society as a whole, to overcoming the view of early education and work–life balance as a "matter for working women". Faced with the challenge of social exclusion, effective early education and work–life balance policies are also an antidote to poverty, as they enable more people from working- and middle-class families to balance and maintain their jobs, instead of being forced to reduce their working day or to abandon their job in order to give care, thereby creating a network of protection for all families.

Governments need to consider well-remunerated leave, early-education policies, and flexible work agreements as a right of "co-responsibility with caregiving" that should be compatible with a socially responsible labor market (Campillo Poza, 2019). These policies do not only benefit families. It is a right for all women and men at different moments of the life cycle, which meets the needs of all generations and improves employment conditions, early-education policies, and labor well-being, and the productivity of all businesses and institutions that have measures to guarantee work–life balance. The aging of the population and gender inequality are pressing challenges in European societies that require a combination of ambitious policies, including (a) equitable assisted reproduction, (b) work–life balance, and (c) early-childhood education and childcare. These would guarantee the co-responsibility of society as a whole in the face of these challenges, and commit institutions to social cohesion as a fundamental pillar of national projects. There is a need for governments to take a lead in providing integrated solutions that harmonize the actions of different states facing these challenges in order to achieve a more just and sustainable society, as well as economic growth.

References

Ahmed, S. (2014). *The cultural politics of emotion*. Edinburgh: Edinburgh University Press.

Audickas, L., & Cracknell, R. (2020). *Social background of MPs 1979–2019*. Number CBP 7483, 27 March 2020. The House of Common Library. Retrieved from https://commons library.parliament.uk/research-briefings/cbp-7483/

Bacchi, C. L., & Goodwin, S. (2016). *Poststructural policy analysis: A guide to practice*. Thousand Oaks: Sage.

BOE. (2006). Boletín Oficial del Estado. Ley 14/2006, de 26 de mayo, sobre técnicas de reproducción humana asistida. BOE-A-2006-9292. Retrieved from www.boe.es/eli/es/l/2006/05/26/14/con

Borraz, M. (2021). El Gobierno Recupera la Reproducción Asistida para Mujeres Lesbianas y sin Pareja e Incluye a las Personas trans (The government restores assisted reproduction for lesbian and single women and includes trans people) *Eldiarioes*. Retrieved from www.eldiario.es/sociedad/gobierno-recupera-reproduccion-asistida-mujeres-lesbianas-pareja-e-incluye-personas-trans_1_8460673.html

Bravo-Moreno, A. (2021). Reproductive agency, assisted reproductive technology & obstetric violence. *Health Care for Women International*. https://doi.org/10.1080/07399332.2021.1883026

Bravo-Moreno, A. (2022). Demystifying the academy: Resistance, ethics and abuse of power. *Power and Education*, *14*(2), 140–156. https://doi.org/10.1177/17577438211068283

British Pregnancy Advisory Service (BPAS). (2015). What's the problem with older mothers? Retrieved from www.bpas.org/get-involved/campaigns/briefings/older-mothers/

Broclchain, M. N., & Beaujouan, E. (2012). Fertility postponement is largely due to rising educational enrolment. *Population Studies, 66*, 311–327. https://doi.org/10.1080/00324728.2012.697569.

Calzada, I., & Brooks, B. (2013). The myth of mediterranean familism: Family values, family structure and public preferences for state intervention in care. *European Societies, 15*(4), 514–534. Retrieved from www.tandfonline.com/doi/abs/10.1080/14616696.2013.836402

Campillo Poza, I. (2019). Políticas de conciliación de la vida laboral, personal y familiar en la Unión Europea [Policies for reconciling work, personal and family life in the European Union] Informes UNAF. Unión de Asociaciones Familiares. Ministerio de Sanidad, Consumo y Bienestar Social. Retrieved from https://unaf.org/wp-content/uploads/2019/10/Informe-UNAF-Poli%CC%81ticas-de-conciliacio%CC%81n-en-la-Unio%CC%81n-Europea.pdf

Castro, C. (2020). Así Perviven las Desigualdades que Legitiman la Violencia Contra las Mujeres Público. November 24. Retrieved from www.publico.es/sociedad/colegio-juzgados-perviven-desigualdades-legitiman-violencia-mujeres.html

Conde-Ruiz, J. I., & Marra de Artinano, I. (2016). Gender gaps in the Spanish labor market. *Estudios sobre la Economía Española, 32,* 1–103. Retrieved from https://documentos.fedea.net/pubs/eee/eee2016-32.pdf

Correll, S. J., Bernard, S., & Paik, I. (2007). Getting a job: Is there a motherhood penalty? *American Journal of Sociology, 112*(5), 1297–1339. Retrieved from https://sociology.stanford.edu/sites/g/files/sbiybj9501/f/publications/getting_a_job-_is_there_a_motherhood_penalty.pdf

Cory, G., & Stirling, A. (2015). Who is breadwinning in Europe. A comparative analysis of maternal breadwinning. Institute for Public Policy Research. Retrieved from www.ippr.org/files/publications/pdf/whos-breadwinning-in-europe-oct2015.pdf

Crawford, S., Boulet, S. L., Mneimneh, A. S., Perkins, K. M., Jamieson, D. J., Zhang, Y, & Kissin, D. M. (2016). Costs of achieving live birth from assisted reproductive technology: A comparison of sequential single and double embryo transfer approaches. *Fertility and Sterility, 105*(2), 444–450. Retrieved from https://doi.org/10.1016/j.fertnstert.2015.10.032

Daily Telegraph. (1981, 16 October). Speech at Conservative Party Conference, 15 October 1981. Daily Telegraph. Retrieved from www.telegraph.co.uk

de la Rica, S., & Gorjón, L. (2016). The impact of family friendly policies in Spain and their use throughout the business cycle. *IZA Journal of European Labour Studies, 5*(9). https://doi.org/10.1186/s40174-016-0059-010.1186/s40174-016-0059-0

Doepke, M., & Zilibotti, F. (2019). *Love, money, and parenting: How Economics explains the way we raise our kids.* Princeton: Princeton University Press.

Donchin, A. (2004). Integrating bioethics and human rights toward a global feminist approach. In Rosemarie Tong, Anne Donchin, & Susan Dodds (Eds.), *Linking visions: Feminist bioethics, human rights, and the developing world* (pp. 31–56). Maryland: Rowman & Littlefield.

ESHRE. (2017). Cross border reproductive care. Retrieved from www.eshre.eu/Press-Room/Resources

ESHRE. (2018). *Cross border reproductive care: The facts from the ESHRE study.* Strombeek-Bever, Belgium: ESHRE.

Esping-Andersen, G. (1990). *The three worlds of welfare capitalism.* Princeton: Princeton University Press.

European Commission/EACEA/Eurydice. (2019). Key data on early childhood education and care in Europe. Eurydice Report. Publications Office of the European Union.

Retrieved from https://eacea.ec.europa.eu/national-policies/eurydice/sites/default/files/kd_ecec_2019_report_en.pdf

European Institute for Gender Equality. (2021). Retrieved from https://eige.europa.eu/gender-mainstreaming/policy-areas/economic-and-financial-affairs/economic-benefits-gender-equality

European Parliament. (2021). The gender perspective in the COVID-19 crisis and post-crisis period. Retrieved from https://oeil.secure.europarl.europa.eu/oeil/popups/ficheprocedure.do?lang=en&reference=2020/2121(INI)

Eurostat. (2019). Reconciliation between Work and Family Life Labour Force Survey (LFS) ad-hoc Module 2018. Retrieved from https://ec.europa.eu/eurostat/web/products-statistical-reports/-/ks-ft-19-006

Eurostat. (2020). Women are having their first child at an older age. Retrieved from https://ec.europa.eu/eurostat/web/products-eurostat-news/-/DDN-20200515-2

Federici, S. (2012). *Revolution at point zero: Housework, reproduction, and feminist struggle.* Oakland: PM Press.

Ferrera, M. (1996). The "southern model" of welfare in social Europe. *Journal of European Social Policy, 6*, 17–37. https://doi.org/10.1177/095892879600600102

Fledderjohann, J., & Barnes, L. W. (2018). Reimagining infertility: A critical examination of fertility norms, geopolitics and survey bias. *Health Policy and Planning, 33*(1), 34–40. https://doi.org/10.1093/heapol/czx148

García-Lumbreras, S. (2019). What if I can't have children with my own ovules. Dexeus Clinic. Retrieved from www.dexeus.com/blog/en/latest/what-if-cant-have-children-with-my-own-ovules

Garnham, A. (2018). Something needs saying about universal credit and women—It is discrimination by design. Child Poverty Action Group. 17 August. Retrieved from https://cpag.org.uk/news-blogs/news-listings/something-needs-saying-about-universal-credit-and-women-%E2%80%93-it-discrimination

Graham, H., & McQuaid, R. (2014). *Exploring the impacts of the UK government's welfare reforms on lone parents moving into work.* Glasgow: Glasgow Centre for Population Health.

Guillén, A. M., & León, M. (Eds.). (2011). *The Spanish welfare state in European context.* London: Routledge.

Harknett, K., Schneider, D., & Luhr, S. (2020). Who cares if parents have unpredictable work schedules? Just-in-time work schedules and child care arrangements. *Social Problems.* https://doi.org/10.1093/socpro/spaa020

HESA. (2022). Higher Education Staff Statistics: UK, 2020/21. Retrieved from www.hesa.ac.uk/news/01-02-2022/sb261-higher-education-staff-statistics#:~:text=The%20percentage%20of%20female%20professors,33%25%20in%202013%2F14.

Hoorens, S., Gallo, F., Cave, J., & Grant, J. C. (2007). Can assisted reproductive technologies help to offset population ageing? An assessment of the demographic and economic impact of ART in Denmark and UK. *Human Reproduction, 22*(9), 2471–2475. https://doi.org/10.1093/humrep/dem181

Institute for Fiscal Studies. (2017). In-work poverty among families with children. Retrieved from www.ifs.org.uk/uploads/publications/comms/r129_ch5.pdf

Instituto Nacional de Estadística (INE). (2019). Encuesta Continua de Hogares. Retrieved from www.ine.es/dyngs/INEbase/es/operacion.htm?c=Estadistica_C&cid=1254736176952&menu=ultiDatos&idp=1254735572981

Jones, O. (2015). *The establishment, and how to get away with it.* London: Penguin.

Katikireddi, S. V., Molaodi, O. R., Gibson, M., Dundas, R., & Craig, P. (2018). Effects of restrictions to Income Support on health of lone mothers in the UK: A natural experiment study. *The Lancet. Public Health, 3*, e333–e340. https://doi.org/10.1016/S2468-2667(18)30109-9

Lawson, V. (2007). Presidential address: Geographies of care and responsibility. *Annals of the Association of American Geographers, 97*, 1–11. www.jstor.org/stable/4620234

León, M., & Migliavacca, M. (2013). Italy and Spain: Still the case of familistic welfare models? *Population Review, 52*(1). https://muse.jhu.edu/article/495518

Lewis, J. (2001). The decline of the male breadwinner model: Implications for work and care. *Social Politics, 8*, 152–169. https://doi.org/10.1093/sp/8.2.152

Lloyd, E. (2015). Early childhood education and care policy in England under the Coalition Government. *The London Review of Education, 13*, 144–156. https://doi.org/10.18546/LRE.13.2.12

López-Casasnovas, G. (2003). *Health care and fiscal decentralisation in Spain*. Barcelona: Universitat Pompeu Fabra. www.upf.edu/documents/2911971/6885257/health_care.pdf/f08632a6-0ce9-4cfd-8f9f-2946d00d2945

Medina, M. Á., & Mateo, J. J. (2019). La Angustia de Pasar años esperando un Tratamiento de Fertilidad en la Sanidad Pública de Madrid (The anguish of spending years waiting for a fertility treatment in the public health of Madrid). *El País*, July 27. Retrieved from https://elpais.com/ccaa/2019/07/26/madrid/1564138816_643498.html

Merrick, R. (2019). Boris Johnson confronted by single mother on live radio show after saying their children are 'ill-raised, ignorant, aggressive and illegitimate'. *The Independent*, November 29. Retrieved from www.independent.co.uk/news/uk/politics/boris-johnson-single-mother-children-spectator-general-election-a9225736.html

Ministerio de Sanidad, Consumo y Bienestar Social. (2020). Tratamientos de Reproducción Asistida en España (Treatments with assisted reproductive technologies in Spain). Retrieved from www.mscbs.gob.es/gabinete/notasPrensa.do?id=5067

Ministerio de Universidades. (2022). Datos y Cifras del Sistema Universitario Español. Publicación 2021-2022. (Facts and Figures of the Spanish University System. Publication 2021-2022). Subdirección General de Actividad Universitaria Investigadora de la Secretaría General de Universidades. https://www.universidades.gob.es/wp-content/uploads/2022/11/Datos_y_Cifras_2021_22.pdf

Naldini, M. (2006). *Le Politiche Sociali in Europa. Trasformazione dei Bisogni Risposte di Policy*. Rome: Carocci.

National Health Service (NHS). (2019). Infertility. Retrieved from www.nhs.uk/conditions/infertility

National Institute for Health and Clinical Excellence (NICE). (2017). Fertility problems: Assessment and treatment. Retrieved from www.nice.org.uk/guidance/cg156 Infertility or www.nhs.uk/conditions/infertility

OECD. (2009). Doing Better for Children. Organization for Economic Co-operation and Development. Retrieved from: www.oecd.org/els/social/childwellbeing

OECD. (2011). Doing better for families. Retrieved from www.oecd.org/social/family/doingbetterforfamilies.htm

OECD. (2020). COVID-19 and key workers: What role do migrants play in your region? OECD COVID-19 Policy Note. Retrieved from www.oecd-ilibrary.org/social-issues-migration-health/covid-19-and-key-workers-what-role-do-migrants-play-in-your-region_42847cb9-en

OECD. (2021). Education GPS. A guide to the OECD social expenditure database. Retrieved from www.oecd.org/social/soc/SOCX_Manuel_2019.pdfOECD

Pickavance, N. (2020). In-work poverty affects many key workers—Now is the time to tackle it. The Financial Inclusion Alliance. April 20. Retrieved from www.peoplemanagement.co.uk/voices/comment/in-work-poverty-affects-many-key-workers-now-is-the-time-to-tackle-it#gref

Prats, J. (2012). Tengo derecho al tratamiento de fertilidad? [Do I have the right to access ART treatment?] *El País*. October 20. Retrieved from https://elpais.com/sociedad/2012/10/19/actualidad/1350675283_805811.html

Randall, V. (2011). Childcare policy in the European states: Limits to convergence. *Journal of European Public Policy, 7*, 346–368. https://doi.org/10.1080/13501760050086071

Salama, M., Isachenko, V., Isachenko, E., Rahimi, G., Mallmann, P., Westphal, L. M., Inhorn, M. C., & Patrizio, P. (2018). Cross border reproductive care (CBRC): A growing global phenomenon with multidimensional implications (a systematic and critical review). *Journal of Assisted Reproduction and Genetics, 35*, 1277–1288. https://doi.org/10.1007/s10815-018-1181-x

Sandher, J. (2019). Foreign-born, working dangerously, and earning less: The UK's key workers. Retrieved from https://blogs.lse.ac.uk/politicsandpolicy/key-workers-covid19

Saraceno, C. (2008). *Gender and care: Old solutions, new developments?* RSCAS Distinguished Lectures. RSCAS DL 2008/02. Florence: European University Institute.

Scully, P., McCandless, E., & Abu-Nimer, M. (2010). Gender violence and gender justice in peacebuilding and development. *Journal of Peacebuilding & Development, 5*(3), 3–6. https://doi.org/10.1080/15423166.2010.778744423430

Slaughter, A.-M. (2015). *Unfinished business. Women, men, work and family*. London: Oneworld Publications.

Social Issues Research Centre. (2012). The changing face of motherhood in Western Europe. Retrieved from www.ohchr.org/EN/HRBodies/CEDAW/Pages/CEDAWIndex.aspx

Statista. (2021). Statista Research Department. Average price of residential property in Europe as of September 2020, per country. Retrieved from www.statista.com/statistics/1052000/cost-of-apartments-in-europe-by-city

Talbot, R. (2021). Single parent discrimination research. Retrieved from www.singleparentrights.org/research

The World Bank. (2019). Retrieved from https://data.worldbank.org/indicator/SP.DYN.TFRT.IN?locations=ES

The World Economic Forum. (2016). The global gender gap report. Retrieved from www3.weforum.org/docs/GGGR16/WEF_Global_Gender_Gap_Report_2016.pdf

Turkmendag, I., Dingwall, R., & Murphy, T. (2008). The removal of donor anonymity in the UK: The silencing of claims by would-be parents. *International Journal of Law, Policy and the Family, 22*, 283–310.

UNICEF. (2011). Children's well-being in UK, Sweden and Spain: The role of inequality and materialism. Retrieved from www.unicef.org.uk/publications/ipsos-mori-child-well-being

UNICEF. (2012). Innocenti Report Card 10. Adamson, Peter. Measuring child poverty. New league tables of child poverty in the world's rich countries. Retrieved from www.unicef-irc.org/publications/pdf/rc10_eng.pdf

Vizard, T. (2019). Families and the labour market. Retrieved from www.ons.gov.uk/employmentandlabourmarket/peopleinwork/employmentandemployeetypes/articles/familiesandthelabourmarketengland/2019

Wayne, J. H., & Casper, W. J., Matthews, R. A., & Allen, T. D. (2016). Why having a family-supportive culture, not just policies, matters to male and female job seekers: An examination of work–family conflict, values, and self-interest. *Sex Roles, 75*, 459–475. https://doi.org/10.1007/s11199-016-0645-7

World Economic Forum. (2016). The Global Gender Gap Report. www.weforum.org/publications/the-global-gender-gap-report-2016/

World Health Organization (WHO). (2000). *The World Health Report 2000 – Health systems: Improving performance*. Geneva: World Health Organization.

World Medical Association (WMA). (2006). Statement on assisted reproductive technologies. Retrieved from www.wma.net/policies-post/wma-statement-on-assisted-reproductive-technologies/

Zucker, A. N. (1999). The psychological impact of reproductive difficulties on women's lives. *Sex Roles, 40*, 767–786. https://doi.org/10.1023/A:1018812819260

Zucker, A. N. (2014). Reproductive justice: More than choice. *Analysis of Social Issues & Public Policies, 14*, 210–221. https://doi.org/10.1111/asap.12059

6 Children's education

Does feminism matter?

Introduction

Given the relationship between family life and inequality, how might the raising of children and the educational practices of solo mothers by choice perpetuate or counteract existing inequalities? How do they challenge traditional practices of gender socialization for their children? This chapter grows out of the interdisciplinarity into which women's studies, gender studies, social anthropology, psychology, education, and feminist methodologies converge. From these perspectives, I examine the praxis in the different motherhoods, which can enrich academic knowledge, thus increasing our understanding of this new type of family. Analyzing different motherhoods raises questions about the meaning and implications of this concept, and it is precisely this reason why neither feminism nor feminist theory can ignore the question of motherhood, since it remains an important aspect in the lives of many women, and the decisions over whether, when, and how to be a mother continue to be a decision to contemplate in their lives. It is therefore important to pay heed to the narratives of these women's lives and to represent their needs. Motherhood has become a place where personal actions are political and where sociocultural values are reflected in personal experience and the experience of their offspring. I agree with Rich (1995), Phoenix et al. (1991), O'Reilly (2009), Hill Collins (1994), Mannis (1999), Mohanty (2003), Green (2011), Minh-ha (1986), and Chase and Rogers (2001) in that there is no one, unique, essential experience of women and mothers out of which universal analytical categories can be derived, but that there are multiple experiences and interpretations regarding women's realities. Furthermore, the concept of feminism is multidimensional, and changeable, because feminisms are created by people who analyze their own oppression and that of their context for the purpose of social change. Depending on the person and her circumstances, the meaning and experience of motherhood are varied. They examine and describe the subtle effects of patriarchy, defining the problems that we must confront and evaluating the strategies for change, and these are all central themes in this chapter. Moreover, parents can choose whether to participate in a gendered family that can affect the lives of their children. Parents' choices can generate unequal opportunities for their children, inequalities that the children have not chosen for themselves.

DOI: 10.4324/9781003269755-7

Mothering and gender are closely intertwined: each is a constitutive element of the other. Perhaps because the gendered allocation of mothering appears to flow inevitably from the division based on reproductive function, mothering, more than any aspect of gender, has been subject to essentialist interpretation: seen as natural, universal, and unchanging. Indeed, for most of the 20th century an idealized model of motherhood derived from the situation of the white, middle class has been projected as universal. In this model, responsibility for mothering rests almost exclusively on one woman (the biological mother) for whom it constitutes the primary if not sole mission during the child's formative years (Allen et al., 2013; Brannon, 2016; Glenn & Forcey, 1994). Moreover, in societies like Spain and Britain where gender stereotypes and biases are ubiquitous, children currently learn to adopt "appropriate" gender roles. These attitudes and behaviors are generally learned first in the home and are then reinforced by the child's peers, school experience, internet, and the media. However, the strongest influence on gender role development seems to occur within the family setting, with parents passing on, both overtly and covertly, to their children their own beliefs about gender (Brannon, 2016). The purpose of this chapter was to bring together interdisciplinary aspects to provide a variety of perspectives on mothering and their views on children's education as a culturally and socially set of practices and relationships involved in nurturing and caring for people; focusing on three themes: (1) the existence of conflict and struggle over competing conceptions of motherhood as an institution and of mothering as an experience; (2) the conditions under which mothering is carried out, and (3) the education of their children.

Family composition and education

Gender is one of the most important pillars upon which sociocultural life is organized (Blakemore et al., 2009). It molds much of a child's identity, it influences the way children are spoken to, how fathers and mothers behave, the opportunities that are offered to them, people's reaction to certain behaviors, leisure interests, and styles of play. According to Blakemore et al. (2009) and (Witt, 1997, p. 253):

> The strongest influence on gender role development seems to occur within the family setting, with parents passing on, both overtly and covertly, to their children their own beliefs about gender. This overview of the impact of parental influence on gender role development leads to the suggestion that an androgynous gender role orientation may be more beneficial to children than strict adherence to traditional gender roles.

A structural characteristic of the family that is particularly relevant for the processes that concern gender is the family composition, that is, in this case, a solo-mother-by-choice family. It is thought that the family make-up, when non-traditional, has an effect in that its members possess fewer traditional attitudes about gender than their families of origin. Biblarz, & Stacey (2010) examined this hypothesis in an extensive review of the literature and concluded that single-motherhood or homosexual parenthood appears to encourage androgynous parenting practices both in mothers and fathers, since these mothers and fathers have to carry out both roles: of provider and carer (Solomon et al., 2005). It seems reasonable to expect that the children from these non-traditional families would adopt fewer traditional values concerning gender. Research on the influence of gender composition in the family is scant and the results varied. However, the available studies (Endendijk, 2015) suggest that gender composition of the family has a direct influence on the behaviors of mothers or fathers in terms of gender. Moreover, there may be a relation between the gender composition of the family (solo mothers, same-sex parents), their behavior, the child's gender cognition, and the child's behavior. The division of gender roles and the paternal or maternal involvement in the family influences this relation, because these gender-related experiences are incorporated into the child's way of thinking about gender, which in turn influence the behavior related to the child's gender. For example, there is evidence that mothers whose own mothers worked outside of the home when they were young had more equitable beliefs about gender than those whose mothers did not (Ciabattari, 2007). The socioeconomic status of the family is also an important factor to consider, since there is ample evidence that shows that it is associated with less traditional attitudes about gender (Bolzendahl & Myers, 2004; Dodson & Borders, 2006; Ex & Janssens, 1998). Moreover, women with higher levels of education have less traditional perspectives on gender than women with less formal education (Harris & Firestone, 1998).

Education also strengthens the belief of both women and men in gender equality (Bolzendahl & Myers, 2004). In fact, paid work, being middle-class, and having a university education are all associated with more egalitarian attitudes for men and women, although this association is stronger in women (Baxter & Kane, 1995). Culture also has a key influence on the gender stereotypes of mothers, fathers, and children through the variations of gender roles in different cultures (Best & Williams, 2001). When gender is an outstanding issue in society, due to its strict division of roles between women and men, these experiences related with gender are likely to be incorporated into the way that society's citizens think about gender (Bem, 1981). I now turn to the thematic analysis revealed through the interpretation of the participants' narratives. For example, the first theme was that of obsolete masculinity, which triggered in the participants the decision to become solo mothers to fulfil their dream to have children. The second theme revolved around how the experience of becoming a solo mother turned into a feeling of empowerment and transgression in relation to the nuclear family. And the third theme developed from the participants' stance on feminism and how different standpoints impact on their children's education and the school they chose. The final phase involved weaving together the analytic narrative and data extracts and contextualizing the analysis in relation to existing literature and the particular context: Spain and Britain. I did thematic analysis by hand with an open coding process (Corbin & Strauss, 1990), identifying data that were related, on a hard copy of the transcripts, by making notes in the margin and by highlighting and giving conceptual labels to sections of text I used the coding to generate themes, building hierarchies of themes which were drawn together from the transcripts to present the findings. My experience as a researcher, in terms of my participation and observation at the research sites, was used to generate a narrative-based interpretation of the events that took place. I present the data from the interviews and observations using quotations from the individual transcripts to illustrate the source of my interpretations (Silverman, 2012).

This study was not driven by a concern for "representativeness". Therefore, it is acknowledged that the sample is not representative of the universe of Spanish or British solo mothers by choice. Kvale (1996, p. 11) states that: "the subject matter [in qualitative research] is no longer objective data to be quantified, but meaningful relations to be interpreted". How widely the discoveries exist in the rest of the world cannot be decided by qualitative methods but by quantitative ones. On the other hand, there may be other self-labels that women adopt, different from the identifications of "feminist" and "non-feminist", that may have yielded other results, and would be worthwhile exploring. However, despite these limitations, this study makes a contribution to the literature and public debates on families, women's life choices, motherhood, and children's education in specific sociocultural contexts that may have an application across societies where women are economically independent. In the next sections, I will analyze the research findings: (a) obsolete versus caring masculinity, (b) emancipatory possibilities of an "alternative" family form, and (c) participants' stance on feminism and how this influences their children's education and school choice.

Analysis of the findings

Obsolete versus caring masculinity

In this section, I will develop two related ideas. First, women who wished to be mothers have opted to be solo mothers because they have not found a suitable partner who will be jointly responsible emotionally and in terms of the childcare and housework that having a family entails. Second, I analyze a type of obsolete masculinity that the participants in this study have condemned and rejected, instead calling for a masculinity that in the literature has been named "caring masculinity" (Scambor et al., 2014). When these women entered adulthood, they believed it would be possible to combine professions in which they would develop their full potential with egalitarian romantic relationships and also parental relationships of joint responsibility. However, none of this study's participants found partners who fulfilled these criteria. As a result, for these women, the cultural and sexual revolutions combined with assisted reproductive technology (ART) converted the idea of maternity outside of the couple as a desirable one. The following quotations sum up the thinking of participants: Cati, 43-year-old mother of a 5-year-old girl, conceived through assisted reproduction, is a Spanish sociologist who currently works in Andalusia (Spain). She defines herself as a feminist.

> I see the brave side, we're pioneers, and this trend is going to become common, as in other European countries … and in that sense, I thought, "why not?" be empowered, take the reins of motherhood, assert that we women can. I have come across some men who, when I say that I'm a solo mother by choice, emphasizing that I have consciously sought to become a mother, have felt bad, rejected. They think: "Ah! This is a radical feminist!" – they also give you the label of radical. Feminism is radical in itself, but even more so. And on top of that, solo mother by choice, they think: "This woman doesn't want men at all!" and they get defensive and say: "You only need our semen. What will this lead to?"

Park et al. (2015) conducted a meta-analysis across six studies to examine men and women interpersonal attraction as a function of shifting features of the environment and they concluded that: "men showed less attraction to women who outperformed them in psychologically near (vs. far) conditions, and this may have been due to decreased feelings of masculinity". Almost a decade earlier Fisman et al. (2006) argued that "in a face-to-face interaction, men found a woman's intelligence appealing up to a point, but once her intelligence outstripped his, his romantic interest waned (…) feelings of diminished masculinity accounted for men's decreased attraction toward women who outperformed them". Another participant, Raquel, is 54 and has a 14-year-old daughter, conceived by assisted reproduction, and another, 9-year-old daughter, through international adoption. She is a journalist and works in a press office in Madrid. She defines herself as a feminist.

> The world of men does not interest me anymore, it's always the same: economic and social power, prestige … The world of women is much more enriching for me, they are more intellectually appealing, they are so much more advanced emotionally … The day that men reach the standard of women, maybe their world will interest me. I am heterosexual, I should have been a lesbian because, well … [she laughs] only one thing interests me in a man … the rest does little for me, emotionally they have brought me very little. I am extremely lucky that my father, my uncles and grandfathers, have given me so much, otherwise it would be terrifying.

Olivia is 43 and has a 4-year-old daughter, conceived through assisted reproduction. She is a psychologist and social worker, and currently works for an NGO in Madrid. She defines herself as a feminist.

> The relationships I have had with men led me to think that having a partner was going to be very difficult. I would have liked to have my daughter with a partner, but with an egalitarian partner, that would be ideal, but as I saw that ideal so unlikely I decided to have my daughter by myself. I thought, I'm going to separate motherhood from having a partner. If I have a partner one day, I will have one because it is worth it and in the meantime I'm going to be a mother.

Miriam is 53 years old and had her daughter, now 7, by assisted reproduction. She has a Ph.D. in pharmaceutics and works for a hospital in Andalusia. She rejects feminism: "I knew I wanted to be a mother. Time was going by and I saw that I wasn't going to find the right person to be my partner and the father of my child". The ideal of "having an egalitarian partner" that the interviewees refer to, which they have not found in their lives, is a common theme in the romantic history of every one of the participants, and they reinforce their argument with examples of their friends. They emphasize that their friends do not get a fair deal in their relationships, that is, most of their friends take charge of the relationship, of motherhood, of taking care of the children, and of what Eichler (2010, p. 36) defines as housework: "the sum of all physical, mental, emotional and spiritual tasks that are performed for one's own or someone else's household, and that maintain the daily life of those for whom one has responsibility". Cati endorses the idea that men are not on a par with women, as jointly responsible for shared lives as partners outside of the hierarchical and chauvinistic relations that many traditional couples in her milieu establish and accept. These are reflected in the statistics, as I have explored in Chapter 5. Furthermore, the participants emphasize that they have not found a man who "is up to the mark" and that, therefore, it is not worth being with a partner for the purpose of having a biparental family because they would not be able to put up with a chauvinist, who would be a burden that none of the participants was willing to tolerate. They would like to be with men who do not fit this pattern, but that is extremely difficult: those men are the exception that they have not found. This is how Cati sums it up:

> Really, being a feminist means that you don't put up with any old relationship, as it were. I see it in comparison with other mothers who I know have a partner, many of them are about to separate, or they have separated, or they cannot stand their husbands, that's what 80% of my acquaintances would tell you.

Lucía, who is 45, a nurse, has a 4-year-old boy conceived through assisted reproduction, and does not define herself as a feminist, explains it in the following way:

> The women I know who have a partner are almost more overwhelmed than I am, because they take charge of their work, their children, their home, and their husbands are more a burden than a help. The woman is the one who carries the whole load, so at least I don't have the burden of a husband.

Their narratives are evidence of the continuing gender inequalities in tandem with the scant range of possibilities that exist for choosing a partner who will be jointly responsible and equitable. According to these women, what men offer them is obsolete, and they are hopeful that the new generations will revise what they have to give. Friedman (2011) asserts that, despite the fact that in the last four decades the options for women to exit their primary role as mother and wife have expanded substantially, the work–family balance has changed to a far lesser degree. According to Coltrane (1997, 2000), the model of the traditional family continues to reflect social expectations, and Hochschild (1989) refers to this as the "stalled revolution": while women have entered the labor market and the public sphere more, men have not become jointly responsible in the home and in childcare. Attitudes towards gender are changing, but experiences in the home are not changing at the same rate. In particular, women are expected to get married or have a partner and take on the greater part of the responsibility for housework and childcare, while men are still expected to fulfil their role as breadwinner, as the statistics from Spain and the United Kingdom show. Women's attitudes have changed at a faster rate than men's, who have been left behind with respect to the levels of joint responsibility in gender equality. The trends in the attitudes of the population reflect that women's entry into the labor market has been supported only to the extent that it has not altered the gender gap in housework and childcare (Conde-Ruiz, J. I. & Marra de Artíñano, 2016; Correll, Benard, & Paik, 2007; van Egmond et al., 2010).

However, there are studies that show that a caring masculinity is emerging as a central way for the future (Scambor et al., 2014). In some cases this is already a reality, along with an increase in the education of women and professional roles, and the rise in expectations over a gender balance in housework and childcare. The results from the education of the mother were the most consistent, as is shown in the literature: the education of women can contribute to the development of more equitable sons. The results of these studies suggest that the experiences and structures around men and boys as well as women and girls must change so that they live and learn gender equality in their local context. Alongside changing policies and structures, we need to deconstruct the unequitable attitudes and norms that many adults and children continue to internalize regarding gender roles and power (Levtov et al., 2014). In the next section, the second central theme developed from the data will be examined: for these women the decision to be solo mothers by choice is transgressive and emancipatory in regard to the traditional nuclear family.

Emancipatory possibilities of an "alternative" family form

Given the unequal nature of heterosexual relations for the participants, the transition to motherhood by themselves has, according to them, brought about an experience of empowerment and emancipation, enabling them to fulfil their wishes to be mothers and to provide their children with positive models of motherhood. Their experience of asymmetrical gender roles with their ex-partners gave rise to the decision to be solo mothers by choice. Vicky, a 54-year-old lawyer who lives in Andalusia and has a 10-year-old son conceived by assisted reproduction, comments thus on her feelings:

> I am used to doing things on my own like travelling, moving from one city to another to find a job … I have a profession, I earn money, I have a mortgage … I feel I have freedom of choice in my life. The fact of having a child on my own was a big step further in fulfilling my dream of becoming a mother, knowing that I would be the main provider for my child felt emancipatory.

Carla, who is 42 and works in human resources for an international company in Madrid, has a 4-year-old daughter conceived through assisted reproduction. She stated:

> I loved the fact of not having to argue with a partner over how to educate my child, the choice of school, ethical values, or who is washing the dishes. I know it's a huge responsibility, if things go wrong, I am the only one to blame! (she laughs). But it's worth it!

For the women in this study, the independence and the apparent increase in possibilities that they experience in their lives are emancipating. All the solo mothers I interviewed considered their motherhood as empowerment, as being in control of their lives, of their own fertility, of their finances, of the education of their children, and of all their family decisions. This was a role that traditionally belonged exclusively to the man, particularly in the era under which many of their families of origin lived. Empowerment appears as an ideal state in which these women are, ultimately, those who exercise control over the factors that affect their lives. Empowerment should have the purpose of challenging and transforming the structures and institutions that reinforce and perpetuate gender discrimination. Jayaweera (1999) posed the question of whether education, in general, empowers women to take control of their lives in a society that reinforces and perpetuates the unequal distribution of power between men and women. Participants' accounts show gender inequalities that are in line with the theories of detraditionalization (Beck & Beck-Gernsheim, 1995; Giddens, 1992), which argue that individualization and life as experimentation are essential. Heelas (1996, p. 2) defines detraditionalization as "a shift of authority: from 'without' to 'within'". It involves the decline in belief in a natural order of established things. While Giddens and Beck are optimistic, as they understand that detraditionalization will bring greater options, opening and reflectiveness, thereby weakening the subjection of old hierarchies, Heelas (1996) argues that parallel processes can exist in a society in which detraditionalization coexists in some aspects at the same time as the traditional is maintained or reconstructed in others (El-Ojeili & Hayden, 2006; Morris, 1996). In this respect, although all the women felt empowered and transgressive in their choice of becoming solo mothers, in the case of half of the sample, that feeling coexisted with their rejection of the feminist label and their decision to choose Catholic or Anglican schools for their children. They chose these schools because, according to them, they taught moral values, therefore maintaining tradition. The other half of the sample interviewed, who defined themselves as feminists, explained what this meant for the education of their children.

Feminist participants, their children's education and school choice

When I asked participants the questions: "What do you think about feminism? Do you consider yourself a feminist?" The answer in half of the sample was a rotund "yes", and they immediately described why: "to create an equal society" or "to provide people with the freedom of choice", for example. They chose secular state schools for their children and they viewed comprehensiveness and inclusiveness as attributes of state schooling. Sonia, who is 51 years of age and lives in Madrid, works for an NGO, and has an 8-year-old daughter conceived through assisted reproduction, explains:

> I wanted a state school for my daughter. I believe in public schooling and public healthcare. We, as citizens, are responsible for paying our taxes and we also have the right to access quality state education and healthcare. I believe in a state school that is inclusive of colors, faiths, socioeconomic backgrounds, genders, abilities, everything that my daughter sees in society and will find in her adult life, when she works in different work environments. I do not believe in elitist, private schools or Catholic schools whose purpose is to indoctrinate children. In those schools there is no room for children of minorities, immigrants and special needs … I fully support state schools, it's a matter of democratic principles.

In Spain, it is the state that currently finances almost all compulsory education. A significant part of the current educational system is private only in the sense that this refers to ownership but not with respect to its sources of funding. Therefore, we can distinguish between state schools (state owned and state funded), grant-maintained schools (privately owned and publicly funded), and private schools (privately owned and privately funded) with a clear predominance of the first over the second and of the second over the third, which constitutes a tiny exception in the range of Spanish education. Spain tops the list of the most state-subsidized private school places in Europe. The Catholic church controls around six out of every ten state-subsidized private schools through the organization "Catholic Schools", which makes it the most representative body of this sector (Escuelas Católicas, 2018). Alberta, from Andalusia, is a lawyer, 47 years of age, and has an 8-year-old boy conceived through assisted reproduction, states that:

> It cannot be denied that an important aim of education is its ability to facilitate social mobility and economic success, although there is little doubt that there are inefficiencies in the state-school system that need to be straightened. However, it is important to understand that the historical and ongoing struggles to provide equal education to women, minorities and special needs demonstrate that state education has been about more than just providing access to the educational conditions needed to secure a job.

Along the same lines, Lola from Madrid, who is 55, a medical doctor with a 10-year-old daughter conceived through assisted reproduction, asserts: "State education and public healthcare are also about the democratic need to value human dignity in advancement of democracy". Therefore, half of the sample thinks that state education in a democracy is much more than just an instrumental means to an economic end; it is also an ethical pillar upon which the structure of democracy rests. Rita, who is 53 and works for a law firm in Madrid, has a 9-year-old daughter conceived through assisted reproduction, and she explains what it means for her to choose a state school for her daughter:

> I chose a state school because I don't like private schools. Firstly, private schools hire teachers endogenously: it is through contacts that people get to teach in private schools. To work at a state school, you need to pass a state examination, they study years before they are able to pass that exam. I did not choose a Catholic school either because I don't want my children to be indoctrinated. I talk to my children about the history of religions, Islamic, Christian, Judaic, and others, but I do not indoctrinate them; when they are older they may choose whatever they want. And thirdly, I think it's about being lucky, regardless of whether it is a private or a state school there are good and bad teachers in both, so I prefer my children to mingle with students from all sorts of backgrounds and to support state schools by sending my children there.

Schools are viewed by these women not only as institutions that impart certain knowledge and skills to students but also as environments that socialize them. They believe that education is a democratizing force that helps to prepare students to participate actively in all aspects of democratic life, imparting the ability to think critically, commitment to democratic values, as well as the basic need to be able to write, read, and do arithmetic. These women have a desire to actively participate in political life, for example, by engaging in school decision-making processes and participating in school parents' associations. In a sense, according to these participants, schools that best teach students the skills to participate actively in democracy are themselves institutions that reflect democratic principles not only in word but also in practice. Therefore, half of the sample thinks that participatory and democratic state school culture makes a significant difference in some of the key building blocks of social responsibility. Ania, who is 43, a teacher in Andalusia, and has a 5-year-old son conceived through assisted reproduction, talks about how it is more likely that state schools put critical pedagogy into practice:

> State schools are in a better position than private or subsidized Catholic schools to reject racism and other forms of discrimination in schools and society fostering pluralism: gender, ethnic, religious, linguistic, economic, etc … that teachers, communities and students reflect. Multicultural education uses critical pedagogy as its philosophy and focuses on social change, therefore trying to promote democratic principles of social justice.

These women thus believed that state schools were better suited for the education they wanted for their children. They view educators and parents as agents who have the potential to develop a social conscience orientated towards justice, recognizing that all knowledge is political, value-laden, and contested, and which should be open to criticism. Educators' beliefs and assumptions about social justice are not immune from questioning. These women also talked about how textbooks are a main source of gender stereotyping. Tania, who is 49 years old, works as a teacher, and has a 9-year-old boy conceived through assisted reproduction, states: "Textbooks all include a lot of gender stereotypes. They are filled with discriminatory representations". Another participant, Silvia, a 42-year-old teacher in Andalusia, says that there is also room for improvement in state teachers' training. She sends her seven-year-old daughter to a state school and describes one incident that took place there:

> For Father's day, my daughter's teacher told her pupils to draw a picture of their dad and to comment on what they liked most about him. Then the teacher displayed all the children's comments on a board outside the classroom. When I went to pick up my daughter I started reading the comments and realised that my daughter's comments were nowhere. I asked her teacher: "Didn't my daughter say anything?" And she replied: "Oh yes, she said wonderful things about you". And I asked her: "Why didn't you include her comments on the board?" And the teacher replied: "Oh, well, it was Father's day … not Mother's day … ". To which I replied: "Your school mission statement says that you are committed to a diverse and inclusive school. Don't you think that by ignoring my daughter's comments, she may have felt excluded due to the fact that she has a different type of family than the nuclear one?" The teacher kept silent and blamed her assistant for not taking into account that my daughter "didn't have a dad".

To manage being a unique family in a social milieu that privileges heterosexual nuclear families raising children, these mothers made a point of educating family members and their schools. Women who perceived that their environment did not support their decision to conceive children as solo mothers by choice worked to help them understand the prejudice and discrimination against this type of families. Silvia, after reflecting on what happened with her daughter, found a children's book entitled: "Tengo una mamá y punto" ("I've got one mum and that's that"). This was a story of a little girl whose family is formed by her mum and her dog. At Silvia's daughter's school, parents could go any Friday to read a story to their children's classroom. Silvia therefore went to read the story of "I've got one mum and that's that", and explained that children have different types of families. The purpose was for the children, their parents, and the teacher to reach a place of acceptance towards her daughter's family formed by a solo mother, so that her family would become just another family in the larger context of different types of families. Laura is also representative of this half of the sample. She is a 45-year-old psychologist and has a 5-year-old daughter, conceived through assisted reproduction. To the question, "How do you apply feminism in the education of your daughter?" she answered:

> I use gender-neutral language when I read stories, I speak with inclusive language to make girls and women visible. I choose books and films that avoid

> gender stereotyping, and it surprises me that she is picking it up and using it. I speak a lot with her about what happens in class. I try to make her see that girls are as capable as boys. And the other day, she told me that she had a fight with some girls in her class because they said that two women could not get married … and I had explained that they could. When we arrived at her classroom, she said to me, Mum, let's go over to the girls: "Isn't it true that two women can get married and can be mothers?" and I explained to her friends that they could, and they were surprised. I consider that educating my daughter in feminism via the premises of social justice, equality and social transformation … means that not only can I support social change but my daughter too. I think it's important that she is aware of this from a young age and that she takes it on as a value from the beginning.

With the awareness that their children would be confronted with questions and prejudices about their family structure or other types of family that did not conform with the heterosexual nuclear family, these feminist mothers also chose to educate their children in order to prepare them for other people's reactions. They thought it was important to educate their children about issues of social justice, for example, by attending different demonstrations with their children, such as the Women's Day March, the march for women's abortion rights, or demonstrations in favor of more funding for state education or state healthcare. In the case of the half of the study sample who see themselves as feminists, motherhood becomes a place of political activism wherein motherhood is consciously fused with their feminism. They take issue with patriarchal ideology in institutions – the family, school, the labor market, and work–family balance policies – practicing alternative forms of motherhood in their way of educating their children. This thus confirms what Horowitz (2004) maintains about feminist mothering as a process of resistance that involves taking decisions about the practice of motherhood. All these women put critical pedagogy into practice as a tool for their children to become aware of social inequality. Critical pedagogy originated with Paulo Freire (1968), who understood education as a political act and asserted that social justice and democracy are not distinct from teaching and learning. The aim of critical pedagogy is emancipation from oppression through an awakening of critical consciousness, defined by Freire as a state of in-depth understanding about the world (1968). "At a fundamental level, to be critically conscious, a child must be a freethinker able to perceive and analyze the world around them as well as any arising contradictions. This in turn leads to the development of social consciousness" (Giroux, 2009, p. 32). Bleazby (2004) suggests that employing critical pedagogy improves a child's academic success, and that implementing critical pedagogy in a mainstream school setting would teach children and adolescents how to think critically about the world that surrounds them, about social dilemmas, the injustices they experience, and how to think, speak, and act better with the purpose of contributing to change to improve society. However, although many of the elements of critical pedagogy can be successfully put into practice in alternative types of education, the practice may be inherently in conflict with mainstream education (Carbonell, 2015). The next section will look into the narratives of the other half of the sample who rejected the feminist label and supported Roman Catholic moral values or Anglican moral values by sending their children to Roman Catholic schools or Anglican schools.

Non-feminist participants and patriarchal beliefs

When I asked these participants, "What do you think of feminism?" some of the answers were: "I do not consider myself a feminist, women are not better than men" and "we should not treat women differently than men, just because they are women". In the case of the women in this study who do not label themselves as feminist, they support some of the attitudes and values of the self-labelled feminist participants, for example, the rejection of obsolete masculinity examined earlier. They also support the economic and social independence of women. The profile of these solo mothers by choice, university-educated professionals, do not need their maternity legitimized by a man within a nuclear family, and they assert that they have created their own practices of motherhood that are, according to them, far from those they were taught in their nuclear families of origin. However, they reject the feminist label as they feel their identities are challenged or contradicted by it. The empowering and emancipatory aspect of being a solo mother by choice for these women coexists with patriarchal ideas about women in society. A case in point is Mila, who is 54 years old, has a Ph.D. in biology, is the head of a hospital department, and has a 7-year-old daughter. I asked her what she thought about feminism, and she responded:

> I don't have a very clear concept of feminism as such … I don't consider myself a feminist … because I don't think that we should stress these differences with men either. Neither men nor women are worse, each one has to carry out the role assigned to them at any given moment as naturally as possible.

Feminism is here viewed as an attempt to upset the "proper" way women and men should act. I was surprised that Mila made no criticism of the sexist education that she herself had acknowledged in her family of origin, with the unequal treatment her parents gave her sister and her compared with their brother. When I asked Mila if she saw anything lacking in social policies, she answered:

> Yes, in the labor sphere, single mothers do not have rights … I have been lucky that my colleagues did not insist on me being on 24-hour call … otherwise I would have had to be on call after my daughter turned one. And I would have had to get by, living alone in this city, and find someone to stay with my daughter. It seems unfair to me, to have to leave a one-year-old child with someone who is not family – what do you really know what that person might do with your child?

Ana: And what did the unions say when you consulted them?

> Mila: That there was no case precedent in law, that nobody had made this type of complaint, and that I could do so, but they didn't know how it would end up, spending my money with no guarantee of what I would achieve.

Despite acknowledging: (a) the unequal treatment in her family of origin, (b) the lack of policies of work–family balance in her job, and (c) the burden borne by her female friends whose husbands did not take joint responsibility of their children and housework, she does not relate any of it to the existing structural inequalities between men and women in society. Rhode (1997, p. 13), speaking of the denial of gender inequality, explains: "And when all else fails, we fall back on biological excuses for sex-based inequalities. Since men and women just are different, we cannot expect society to equalize their status". Monique's arguments regarding the difference between men and women in society reinforces the idea that is due to biological differences. Monique, a Belgian physiotherapist, who is 53 and Catholic, arrived in London 25 years ago and used her own eggs and sperm from a donor at a private clinic in London. She started with ART at the age of 37 and after seven attempts over a five year period she had her son who is now 10. Regarding feminism, Monique states that:

> I'm not a feminist or someone who is going to campaign for feminism or anything like that. I think you just have to live in accordance with what you believe, and if you do that you show people by doing rather than by saying and campaigning. It's good that some women do it, because there are obviously some problems … feminism, racism.

It is interesting that Monique says that one of the problems is "feminism". It may have been a mistake, although she did not notice. Rhode (1997, p. 14) argues that "women working a double shift at home and on the job are generally reluctant to take time for political action". When we talked about children's education and challenging stereotypes, Monique explained that: "obviously there is a difference between males and females I do believe that our bodies express something that comes from inside and I think that's why males and females are different". Non-feminist participants hold the belief that biology is equally or even more significant than culture in shaping "masculine" and "feminine" characteristics. These misconceptions contribute to the failure of these women to recognize gender inequality as a significant issue.

Whatever their biological predispositions, children receive strong cultural signals about gender-appropriate tasks and behaviors. Much of their learning comes from unintended or indirect messages. If, as is still the case, parents assign more homemaking chores to daughters than to sons, children will learn what is "women's work". Research conducted in 2023 among 4,010 UK adults in a heterosexual relationship concluded that women were primarily responsible for 10 of the 14 tasks analyzed, while men were responsible for 4. The division of different chores also followed entrenched gender stereotypes. The task of cleaning, for example, was five times more likely to fall on women's shoulders than men's (52% vs. 10%), in addition to tidying (49% vs. 10%). Women were also six times more likely to do the laundry (62% vs. 10%). Gender stereotypes worked both ways. Men were more likely to take responsibility for tasks that took place outdoors, and were 12 times more likely to look after car maintenance (74% vs. 6%), and more than twice as likely to be responsible for gardening (47% vs. 20%) (Mortar Research, 2023).

Another significant and representative case of this half of the sample is Daniela, 47-year-old managing director of one of the largest shopping centers of a city in Spain, who holds an MBA, and has a 6-year-old son, conceived through assisted reproduction. She told me that in her previous job, for a company in Madrid, they did not renew her contract because she was pregnant. Daniela excused the company because "pregnant women cause a company losses", implying that women's choices explain women's disadvantages in an attempt to justify that inequality (Rhode, 1997, p. 9). Today, as the managing director of a shopping center, she states:

> Women have a bad name in companies, but it's that, sometimes, it's true. In this company there are women who have used their pregnancy to get sick leave, and pregnancy is not an illness, what they have is a lot of cheek.

This quotation makes sense in light of the Queen Bee phenomenon (Ellemers et al., 2012), whereby "Queen Bees" are senior women in masculine organizational cultures who have fulfilled their career aspirations by dissociating themselves from their gender while simultaneously contributing to the gender stereotyping of other women. They implicitly legitimize rather than question the disadvantaged position of women within their organization and perpetuate the organizational culture in which they became successful. Later in the interview talking about her male colleagues, Daniela recognizes that:

> Men have everything much easier: they leave their children with their wife and can work as many hours as they like, then they get home to food on the table and the children already ready for bed.

As I explained earlier, in Spain and in the United Kingdom women are often responsible for restructuring hours to accommodate family needs. Despite her assertion, Daniela does not see the need for feminism and criticizes positive action, such as measures targeted at women to readdress discriminations or to offset disadvantages arising from existing attitudes, behaviors, and social structures in the companies she used to work for and at her present company. Another participant, Sandra, a 50-year-old pharmacist from Andalusia, who has a 5-year-old son conceived through assisted reproduction, invited me to join an outing with four heterosexual couples and two solo mothers by choice with the help of ART, along with our children, who were aged between four and ten. I described my observations in my fieldwork diary:

> We went to a restaurant, and children and adults were going to sit at different tables. When the adults were about to sit at their table Sandra almost shouted: "Please let the men go to that part of the table and we (women) can sit here, nearer the play area so that we can check on the kids".

Through this statement, Sandra, who claims to be independent and empowered by becoming a solo mother, differentiates the role men and women play in families and reproduces representations of femininity and masculinity, such as independence as opposed to "feminine" qualities attributed to the ideal mother: dedication to the family, care and sacrifice for her children (and husband). Similarly, I wrote in my field notes about Nadia's comments to her son. Nadia is a 54-year-old entrepreneur from Madrid, and her son, who is 9, was conceived through assisted reproduction. During our interview her son started crying because he had fallen to the ground, and once she had seen that his wound was superficial, she said to him: "you are a big boy, people are going to think you are like a little girl". The message that this boy is receiving about what it means to be male is limiting and stereotypical. This message may also come from peers, the media, and elsewhere, telling boys and men how to behave and feel, relate to each other and girls and women, and what their role and importance is in society. Nadia is not aware that when boys are taught to act a certain way, to oppose qualities traditionally viewed as "feminine", gender stereotypes may contribute to gender differences. However, for these women it seems that the responsibility for perpetuating the cycle of sexism lies elsewhere. In general, despite the fact that these participants reject feminism, they benefit from the advances of the feminist movement, such as the right to vote, the right to contraception, the right to abortion, and the right to divorce. In particular, these women have made use of the progressive Law 35/1988 (BOE, 1988) and Law 14/ 2006 (BOE, 2006) on assisted reproduction, which brought about a technical and scientific advance on the legislation of neighboring countries (France, Germany, the United Kingdom, and Italy). These laws are still a benchmark, both for the techniques that it regulates and for those who can use them independent of their civil status and sexual orientation, and it allows the use of assisted reproduction not only for fertility problems but to postpone motherhood with own or others' oocytes, and as an option to create a solo-mother family. In the case of these participants, it might be thought that the women's choice to be solo mothers, their financial independence, and their university education, all of which nourish their perception of empowerment, would mean that they participated in feminist practices. However, they rarely attributed the imbalance of power between men and women in contexts of work, family, or friends, to inequality (Blasco,2018). Rawat (2014), in her study on patriarchal beliefs, women's empowerment and general well-being, concludes that educational level, professional success, and economic independence do not have an impact on patriarchal beliefs. Yoon et al. (2015) conducted a quantitative study based on a sample of American women and identified three correlated factors of the patriarchal beliefs scale: modern sexism (i.e., covert and subtle sexism), antifeminist attitudes, and some egalitarian attitudes (vs. traditional attitudes) towards women. Sample items included "economic and social freedom is worth far more to women than acceptance of the ideal of femininity which has been set up by men" (p. 270). Jackman (1994), Jost and Banaji (1994), and Sidanius and Pratto (1999) argue that subordinate groups often contribute to their own subordination by accepting the ideology of the dominant group as valid. Furthermore, Bhasin and Khan (1999) state that feminism is an awareness of patriarchal control, exploitation, and oppression from an ideological and material context of women's work, fertility, sexuality, family, the labor market, and society in general, and needs conscious action by women and men to transform the present situation. Gender consciousness is the extent to which one interprets experiences through a gendered lens (Gurin & Markus, 1989). Nevertheless, these participants lack that awareness or gender consciousness, denying either that gender inequality is a serious problem or that it is one that they have a personal or political responsibility to address.

Non-feminist participants and their children's education

When I asked these women: "When you and your child watch cartoons, films or read stories in which gender stereotypes normally exist, do you analyze them with your child?" Eva, a 48-year-old Spanish lawyer with an 8-year-old son, who defines herself as a non-feminist, epitomizes the thinking of these participants:

> My son lives with me in an environment where there are women who are the breadwinners, who are strong. My sister is a doctor [she says "médico" instead of "médica", using the traditional, masculine word to describe her sister's profession, which shows that she continues to reproduce linguistic sexism]. My son is often around my female workmates, many of whom run their homes alone with their children. Perhaps I have not started to explain him things in a proactive way. I think that, little by little, he is becoming imbued with this … that … well, that women are just as strong as men and can do the same things …

Liz, 47, white British, heterosexual, director of a research company in London, explained that she would have loved to have been part of a couple, but she never found someone to be part of a couple with so, she found herself in the situation where ART was the only way to become a mother, other than adopting a child. At the hospital they did an ovarian reserve test, the results came back showing very poor quality eggs and the doctor said to her: "don't waste your money, you've got a nano percentage chance". Then her sister asked her: "why don't I give you some of my eggs?" She was told that there was a real shortage of UK sperm donors and bought sperm from a sperm bank in the United States, had IVF procedure over 4 years and paid £30,000, then she got pregnant with her son who is two and a half years old. When I asked her about feminism, she stated:

> I'm not a very ideological person so I don't consider myself a feminist in a political sense, but I totally believe in equal rights for women. I went to an all-girls school from the age of eight and I left school believing that I could do anything.

Nevertheless she points out the sexism she encountered in her previous job:

> Funnily enough, in the last few years I've encountered a sexism at work, which none of the men in the room would've seen or would've believed, and would have been horrified if I'd said to them, "don't patronize me in that way". I was on a management board with a group of men and I just felt patronized so much of the time. I felt like, "I've got better ideas than you, you're all just posing in front of each other" it's such an unproductive working environment. They were all too busy loving the sound of their own voices ... I think I probably am a feminist but I wouldn't really label myself as one, if that makes sense.

And when I asked her how does she translate that non-labelled feminism into the education of her child Liz describes that she and her son go to an Anglican Church every Sunday because there is "a really nice school attached to that Church" and potentially try and get her son to that school. If they attend Church a consistent number of times, according to the vicar, her son will be able to enroll in that school, which costs £1,500 a month. Liz explains that:

> The vicar, who's a lady in the church where my son was christened, came round my home for a cup of tea to talk about the christening, and she said: "by the way if you're worried about being a single mother, I have baptized hundreds of babies of single mothers, so please don't". Which was really nice. I haven't really run into any problems for being a solo mother and a Christian.

Liz expands on how she educates her son:

> He's got his dollies, he loves his kitchen, but I've not consciously ... I think it's very hard ... he said, "you can have the pink one mummy and I'll have the blue one" ... I remember my niece saying this actually, a load of blue cards arrived for her little brother and she's like, "blue's for boys and pink is for girls, isn't it mummy". She wasn't even three and she'd worked out that pink is for girls and blue is for boys. You can't change the fact that girl cards are pink and boy cards are blue, but you can, sort of, do your bit to, being a working mother, you know him seeing role modelling working, is also important.

Liz uses the same argument as Eva, they are reluctant to be labelled "feminists" but her son and her daughter, respectively, see them working and will one day think that men and women can do the same. Nonetheless, according to Giroux (2009) it is not enough for children to have a "strong" mother who works outside and inside the home, but that an effort must be made to pedagogically explain the injustices and inequalities of power in society so that children are aware of them and do not go on to reproduce them. All these participants chose Christian schools for their children, and all of them stated that "Christian schools teach values". Elsa, who is

45, a judge from Andalusia, and has a 4-year-old daughter, explains why she chose a Catholic school for her daughter:

> At the age of 3 my daughter was singing "Our Father in heaven". They pray every day (she smiled) ... this school will teach her values, at least. Apart from the fact that I may be more or less religious ... I don't go to church every Sunday (she smiled) but I believe in God. I chose it because they say it is a very good school, children start from the age of 3 and can continue up to the age of 18, most children from our apartment block go to that school so it is good for her, and it is easy for me to drive her there. I didn't think of anything else: they were good enough reasons for me.

Patricia, who is 43, a gynecologist from Madrid, and has a 5-year-old son, comments on why she chose a Catholic school:

> I was educated in a Catholic school. I wanted my son to have moral values, self-discipline and an excellent education. I prefer a Catholic school where you know what kind of children get in. I didn't want a ghetto school populated by mostly children of immigrants or by gypsies that could slow the learning of my child. I chose students' selection and moral values.

Jaqueline who is 38, white French, heterosexual, and Catholic, who asserted that she does not care what the Pope thinks about ART. She came to London from France 20 years ago, works in human resources, and earns £100,000 per year and pays £1,700 a month for a childminder for her 3 months old boy. It took her six years to become pregnant. She became pregnant twice but did not result in a baby, and had a double donation: egg donation in London and sperm from a donor bank abroad. She says that she is no gender neutral, she wants her son to "be a boy":

> I'm raising him as a boy, dressing him as a boy. I like it. Traditional ways and expectations, that is, toys wise he will get cars and trucks. If he wants a doll, he will get a doll but I'm not going to be the one who will put it in front of him. He might wear pink, who knows, but otherwise he will be more in boy's colors like blue, green, brown and white.

When toys and colors talk, their messages, both literal and symbolic, support conventional gender stereotypes (Rhode, 1997, p. 19). In the future Jaqueline wants her son to attend an international school, so that he can get a French–English bilingual education for £12,790 per year for primary school. These participants are concerned about the impact of "social mixture" in state schools, which may include children from poor socioeconomic background, children from minority groups, and children of immigrants. They therefore enroll them in private, state-subsidized Catholic schools or Anglican Church schools that are located in middle-class neighborhoods and which provide a more "exclusive" environment. Around the time that the interviews took place, the national news media was discussing the Pope's views on reproductive technologies, which he called into question because they "introduced the ability to manipulate the reproductive act", and on single mothers, stating that "the absence of a father gravely affects family life and the upbringing of children and their integration into society" (Libreria Editrice Vaticana, 2016). At the same time, national news also spoke about allegations of sexism in Catholic schools in Madrid, when a Catholic school was investigated after it emerged that while boys were offered an extracurricular trip to the Real Madrid stadium, girls were offered crochet classes (Galaup, 2017). Indeed, numerous studies demonstrate the relation between sexism and religiosity and the reinforcement of sexist attitudes in the students of religious schools (Glick et al., 2002; Maltby & Hall, 2014; Mikołajczak & Pietrzak, 2014; Seguino, 2011; Stitzlein, 2008). However, none of the Spanish participants knew about the Pope's views on reproductive technologies and solo mothers. Rita, 44 years old, a journalist from Madrid who has a daughter through assisted reproduction, responded: "I didn't know what the Pope thought, but my daughter is very happy in her [Catholic] school, and we were not treated differently because of my being a single mum". Another participant, Ada, who is from Andalusia, is 40 years old, and is a nurse with a 4-year-old daughter by assisted reproduction, remarked: "En todos los sitios cuecen habas" ("we all have something to hide"). In other words, she asserted that there may be sexism anywhere, minimizing the importance of sexism in Catholic schools, as well as the Pope's views on families who do not follow the heterosexual nuclear family structure.

According to Sallam and Sallam (2016) human response to new developments regarding birth is largely shaped by religious beliefs and assisted reproduction is unacceptable to Roman Catholicism, whereas Anglicans accept most of its forms, which do not involve gamete or embryo donation. Tamayo Acosta, professor of theology and the science of religions, argues that religions have a patriarchal structure, transmitting an androcentric ideology, imposing a sexist morality, and developing sexist practices. He alleges that Judaism and Christianity are the basis of Western patriarchy, and that they have been one of the greatest obstacles to women's emancipation (Tamayo Acosta, 2011). Patriarchal structures are internalized as patriarchal beliefs at an individual level. As Yoon et al. (2015, p. 264) explain:

> Patriarchal beliefs are developed through social learning and also serve to reinforce the patriarchal system by informing gendered behaviors and decision making. In spite of increased equality for women as a group, patriarchal beliefs are so deeply engrained in daily lives and social systems that it is often difficult to tease them apart from our consciousness.

The origin of "implicit" prejudice goes back to early childhood: when children learn about the world that surrounds them and neuronal associations are created in the brain that relate concepts and memories in an unconscious manner (Carnes et al., 2015). These associations are cultural, but they are set as pathways in our brain and unconsciously accompany us throughout our lives, and they also predispose us to have prejudices about gender, skin color, religion, and socioeconomic status. In particular, conscious gender bias can begin at the age of 5, but if it is not supported by the environment it can disappear around the ages of 10–12. If these stereotypes are supported by the children's environment, the die is cast. Implicit biases, however, can be developed as young as three years old (Roberts et al., 2016). Once established at preschool age, they can be difficult to change. While conscious biases are not sustained in many children, implicit or unconscious biases normally remain constant throughout adulthood (Johnston, 2017). Bartky (1990, p. 25) argues: "Exposure to stereotypes can cause women to internalize these ideas and believe them, both consciously and unconsciously". For Bourdieu and Wacquant, gender relations are the paradigm case of the operation of symbolic violence, which denotes more than a form of violence operating symbolically. It is "the violence which is exercised upon a social agent with his or her complicity" (Bourdieu & Wacquant, 1992, p. 167). Other authors argue that there is an internalization of sexism to justify the hostility of women towards women (Cowan & Ullman, 2006), or a combination of internalization and subtyping, that is, the Queen Bee phenomenon (Ellemers et al., 2012), to explain women's endorsement of sexist beliefs. Zimmermann and Gygax (2016) suggest that the tendency for some socially shared norms to be interpreted as inevitable may complement these explanations of women's endorsement of sexist beliefs.

Reflections

The emphasis of this chapter was focused on why participants of this study, half of them self-labelled as feminist and the other half as non-feminist, decided to become solo mothers with the help of ART, and on what they experienced, and how their educational choices may challenge traditional practices of gender socialization for their children. All the women interviewed define their motherhood as empowering and transgressive with respect to the traditional nuclear family, and all of them criticize the obsolete masculinity of their former partners and male acquaintances, as well as being hopeful that in future generations obsolete masculinity will be replaced by caring masculinity. However, despite the fact that the literature indicates that family composition, when non-traditional, has an effect because its members possess fewer traditional attitudes about gender than their families of origin, and that women's university education, financial independence, professional success, and belonging to the middle class, can all encourage more egalitarian attitudes, none has brought about a profound change in the patriarchal ideology of the non-feminist participants. These participants hold women accountable for inequality: women's choices explain women's disadvantages. They are uncomfortable with feminism because it threatens their understanding of their identity and worldview. They do not see social structures as contributing to inequality and view positive action measures as mistaken. They lack gender consciousness and deny either that gender inequality is a serious problem or that it is one that they have a personal or political responsibility to confront. They do not have the self-awareness of belonging to a historically discriminated group. This strong resistance points to the systematic historical, cultural, psychological, and structural character of patriarchal organization. As we have seen, different concepts can be applied to this, such as: Bourdieu's symbolic violence; the acceptance of the ideology of the dominant group as valid; the internalization of sexism to justify the hostility of women towards women; or a combination of internalization and subtyping, or the tendency for some socially shared norms to be interpreted as inevitable to explain women's endorsement of sexist beliefs. Johnston (2017) uses the concept of unconscious bias, that is, cultural associations learned in our childhood that predispose us to have prejudices about gender, skin color, religion, and socioeconomic status.

Uncovering the interconnections of the sociocultural network in which these women live and from which they have extracted elements to construct their own identity is no easy task. They reject feminism and have not acquired an awareness that requires actions to transform the present situation. Yet they hope that their children, because they are offspring of solo-mother families, comprehend that both men and women "can do the same things" and have the right to be socially and economically independent. Nonetheless, they show patriarchal beliefs and they have chosen Catholic and Anglican schools, in Spain and Britain, respectively, for their children, a choice that ideologically repeats and perpetuates sexism. Enloe (2017, p. 81) argues that patriarchy "is as current as our contemporary governments, economic systems, and policies. It is adaptive, dynamic, and sustainable, and it is our reluctance to examine patriarchal structures, values, beliefs, and behaviors that enables it to survive". Therefore, change will require active attentiveness, reflection, questioning, and investigation if we want to illuminate how interwoven ideas about sex, gender, and difference are in the world we live in. Conversely, the other half of this study's sample define themselves as feminist. They espouse critical pedagogy in their children's education, exercising critical consciousness focused on attaining an understanding of the world that identifies political, economic, and social contradictions and acting against the oppressive elements in their lives, as well as intervening in the reality that surrounds them with the aim of changing it. Thus, they educate their children in the belief that sex and gender should not determine their place in the world, problematizing and challenging the government for their lack of public policies and mainstream schools for reproducing, in many cases, patriarchal beliefs. They offer alternative family models with the commitment that they can change society and serve as a link so that their children change it in the direction indicated by Feldman Barrett (2017, p. 158): "It's possible for each person to change their concepts and therefore their behavior". These women do not claim that feminism, critical pedagogy, and secular schools are the solution to social inequality.

However, they recognize the inextricable link between personal transformation and social transformation, creating a pathway between their sense of injustice, their actions, and their participation in feminist and social justice movements. The challenge is not simply to encourage change and to criticize systems but to put it into practice. They point to the centrality of gender consciousness in relation to feminist attitudes and political activism. Duncan (2010) shows that feminist identity mediates the relationships between political activism and authoritarianism, education, and experiences with sexism. We cannot change society without changing ourselves, and we cannot change ourselves without recognizing our embeddedness and interconnectedness in sociocultural processes and institutions. Thus, to be able to transform society, it is crucial that families and schools participate in the processes of change, since it is through key institutions such as these, amongst other factors, that patriarchal belief systems are transmitted and reproduced.

References

Allen, K. R., Walker A. J., & McCann, B. R. (2013). Feminism and families. In G. Peterson, & K. Bush (Eds.), *Handbook of marriage and the family* (pp. 139–58). Boston, MA: Springer.

Bartky, S. L. (1990). *Femininity and domination: Studies in the phenomenology of oppression*. New York, NY: Routledge.

Baxter, J., & Kane, E. W. (1995). Dependence and independence: A Cross-national analysis of gender inequality and gender attitudes. *Gender & Society, 9*(2), 193–215.

Beck, U., & Beck-Gernsheim, E. (1995). *The normal chaos of love*. Cambridge, UK: Polity Press.

Bem, S. L. (1981). Gender schema theory: A cognitive account of sex typing. *Psychological Review, 88*(4), 354–364.

Best, D. L., & Williams, J. E. (2001). Gender and culture. In D. Matsumoto (Ed.), *The handbook of culture and psychology* (pp. 195–219). New York, NY: Oxford University Press.

Bhasin, K., & Khan, N. S. (1999). *Some questions on feminism and its relevance in South Asia*. New Delhi, India: Kali for Women.

Biblarz, T. J., & Stacey, J. (2010). How does the gender of parents matter? *Journal of Family and Marriage, 71*(1), 3–22.

Blakemore, J. E., Berenbaum S. A., & Liben L. S. (2009). *Gender development*. New York, NY: Psychology Press.

Blasco, E. (2018, February 2). El 8 de marzo tiene que ser una jornada histórica para acabar con la discriminación, para corregir la desigualdad laboral y social que sufren las mujeres [March 8 has to be a historic day to end discrimination, to correct the labor and social inequality suffered by women]. CCOO. Retrieved from www.ccoo.es/noticia:270383

Bleazby, J. (2004). Practicality and philosophy for children. Critical & creative thinking. *The Australasian Journal of Philosophy in Education, 12*(2), 33–42.

Boletín Oficial del Estado (BOE). (1988). No. 282, Law 35/1988, 22nd of November. Sobre técnicas de reproducción asistida Departmaento Jefatura de Estado [On techniques of assisted reproduction, Department Head of State]. Retrieved from www.boe.es/buscar/doc.php?id=BOE-A-1988-27108

Boletín Oficial del Estado (BOE). (2006). No. 126, Law 14/2006, 27th of May. Sobre técnicas de reproducción humana asistida. Departamento Jefatura de Estado [On techniques of assisted human reproduction, Department Head of State]. Retrieved from www.boe.es/buscar/act.php?id=BOE-A-2006-9292

Bolzendahl, C. I., & Myers, D. J. (2004). Feminist attitudes and support for gender equality: 942 The Qualitative Report 2019 Opinion change in women and men, 1974–1998. *Social Forces, 83*(2), 759–789.

Bourdieu, P., & Wacquant, L. (1992). *An invitation to reflexive sociology*. Chicago, IL: Chicago University Press.

Brannon, L. (2016). *Gender. Psychological perspectives*. New York: Routledge.

Carbonell, J. (2015). La escuela pública no es de los maestros ni del Estado; es de la comunidad [The public school is not of the teachers or of the State; it's from the community]. El Diario [The Newspaper]. Retrieved from www.eldiario.es/1187eminism1187/Jaume-Carbonell-escuela-maestros-comunidad_0_355215521.html

Carnes, M., Devine, P. G., Baier Manwell, L., Byars Winston, A., Fine, E., Ford, C. E., & Sheridan, J. (2015). The effect of an intervention to break the gender bias habit for faculty at one institution: A cluster randomized, controlled trial. *Academic Medicine, 90*(2), 221–230.

Chase, S. E., & Rogers, M. E. (Eds.). (2001). *Mothers and children: Feminist analyses and personal narratives*. New Brunswick, NJ: Rutgers University Press.

Ciabattari, T. (2007). Single mothers, social capital, and work-family conflict. *Journal of Family Issues, 28*(1), 34–60.

Coltrane, S. (1997). *Family man: Fatherhood, housework, and gender equity*. Oxford, UK: Oxford University Press.

Coltrane, S. (2000). Research on household labor: Modeling and measuring the social embeddedness of routine family work. *Journal of Marriage and Family, 62*(4), 1208–1233. Doi.org/10.1111/j.1741-3737.2000.01208.x

Conde-Ruiz, J. I., & Marra de Artíñano, I. (2016). Gender gaps in the Spanish labor market. Madrid, Spain: Fundación de Estudios de Economía Aplicada (FEDEA). Retrieved from www.fundacionalternativas.org/laboratorio/documentos/zoom—economico/brechas-salariales-de-genero-en-espana

Corbin, J., & Strauss, A. (1990). Grounded theory research: Procedures, canons, and evaluative criteria. *Qualitative Sociology, 13*(1), 1–19. https://med-fom-familymed-research.sites.olt.ubc.ca/files/2012/03/W10-Corbin-and-Strauss-grounded-theory.pdf

Correll, S. J., Benard, S., & Paik, I. (2007). Getting a job: Is there a motherhood penalty? *American Journal of Sociology, 112*(5), 1297–1339.

Cowan, G., & Ullman, J. B. (2006). Ingroup rejection among women: The role of personal inadequacy. *Psychology of Women Quarterly, 30*(4), 399–409.

Dodson, T. A., & Borders, D. (2006). Men in traditional and non-traditional careers: Gender role attitudes, gender role conflict, and job satisfaction. *The Career Development Quarterly, 54*(4), 283–296.

Duncan, L. E. (2010). Women's relationship to feminism: Effects of generation and feminist self-labeling. *Psychology of Women Quarterly, 34*, 398–507.

Eichler, M. (2010). What is housework? In M. Eichler, P. Albanese, S. Ferguson, N. Hyndman, L. Liu, & A. Matthews (Eds.), *More than it seems: Household work and lifelong learning* (pp. 21–48). Toronto, Canada: Women's Press.

Ellemers, N., Rink, F. A., Derks, B., & Ryan, M. K. (2012). Women in high places: When and why promoting women into top positions can harm them individually or as a group (and how to prevent this). *Research into Organizational Behavior, 32*, 163–187.

El-Ojeili, C., & Hayden, P. (2006). *Critical theories of globalization: An introduction*. Basingstoke, UK: Palgrave.

Endendijk, J. J. (2015). Heroes and housewives: The role of gender and gender stereotypes in parenting and child development (Doctoral Thesis). Child and Family Studies, Institute of Education and Child Studies, Faculty of Social and Behavioural Sciences, Leiden University. Retrieved from https://openaccess.leidenuniv.nl/handle/1887/32778

Enloe, C. (2017). *The big push: Exposing and challenging the persistence of patriarchy*. Oakland, CA: California of University Press.

Escuelas Católicas. (2018). Estadística [Statistics]. Escuelas Católicas [Catholic Schools]. Retrieved from www.escuelascatolicas.es/estadistica/

Ex, C. T., & Janssens, J. M. (1998). Maternal influences on daughters' gender role attitudes. *Sex Roles, 38*(3–4), 171–185.

Feldman Barrett, L. (2017). *How emotions are made: The secret life of the brain*. Basingstoke, UK: Pan Macmillan.

Fisman, R., Iyengar, S., Kamenica, E., & Simonson, I. (2006). Gender differences in mate selection: Evidence from a speed dating experiment. *Quarterly Journal of Economics, 121*, 673–697.
Freire, P. (1968). *Pedagogía del oprimido*. Madrid, Spain: Siglo XXI.
Friedman, S. D. (2011). Implications of the revolution in work and family. Open Mind. BBVA. Retrieved from www.bbvaopenmind.com/en/articles/implications-of-the-revolution-in-work-and-family/
Galaup, L. (2017, April 30). El colegio denunciado por actividades sexistas y mensajes homófobos recibe dos millones públicos anuales [The school denounced for sexist activities and homophobic messages receives two million public per year]. El Diario [The Newspaper]. Retrieved from www.eldiario.es/1208eminism/educacion_segregada-financiation_publicaComunidad_de+Madrid_0_636936442.html
Giddens, A. (1992). *The transformation of intimacy: Sexuality, love, and eroticism in modern societies*. Stanford, CA: Stanford University Press.
Giroux, H. A. (2009). Critical educational theory and educational practice. In A. Darder, M. Baltodano, & R. D. Torres (Eds.), *The critical pedagogy reader* (pp. 27–55). New York, NY: Routledge Falmer.
Glenn, E. C., Forcey, L.R. (Eds.) (1994). *Mothering: Ideology, experience, and agency*. New York: Routledge.
Glick, P., Lameiras, M., & Castro, C. (2002). Education and Catholic religiosity as predictors of hostile and benevolent sexism toward women and men. *Sex Roles, 47*(9–10), 433–441.
Green, F. J. (2011). *Practicing feminist mothering*. Winnipeg, Canada: Arbeiter Ring Publishing.
Gurin, P., & Markus, H. (1989). Cognitive consequences of gender identity. In S. Skevington, & D. Baker (Eds.), *The social identity of women* (pp. 152–172). Newbury Park, CA: Sage.
Harris, R. J., & Firestone, J. M. (1998). Changes in predictors of gender role ideologies among women: A multivariate analysis. *Sex Roles, 38*(3–4), 239–252.
Heelas, P. (1996). Introduction: Detraditionalization and its rivals. In P. Heelas, S. Lash, & P. Morris (Eds.), *Detraditionalization: Critical reflections on authority and identity* (pp. 1–20). Cambridge, UK: Blackwell.
Hill Collins, P. (1994). Shifting the centre: Race, class, and feminist theorizing about motherhood. In E. Nakano Glenn, G. Chang, & L. Rennie Forcey (Eds.), *Mothering. Ideology, experience and agency* (pp. 45–62). New York, NY: Routledge.
Hochschild, A. R. (1989). *The second shift: Working parents and the revolution at home*. New York, NY: Viking Press.
Horowitz, E. (2004). Resistance as a site of empowerment: The journey away from maternal sacrifice. In A. O'Reilly (Ed.), *Mother outlaws: Theories and practices of empowered mothering* (pp. 43–58). Toronto, Canada: Canadian Scholars' Press.
Jackman, M. R. (1994). *The velvet glove: Paternalism and conflict in gender, class, and race relations*. Berkeley, CA: University of California Press.
Jayaweera, S. (1999). Gender, education, development: Sri Lanka. In C. Herward, & S. Bunwaree (Eds.), *Gender, education and development beyond access to empowerment* (pp. 185–186). London, UK: Zed Books Ltd.
Johnston, I. (2017, February 18). Racism and sexism stem from 'optical illusion' in brain that is 'part of human condition', academic says. Independent Newspaper. Ian Johnston. Retrieved from www.independent.co.uk/news/science/racism-sexismprejudice-implicit-bias-universities-students-graduation-aaas-a7587716.html
Jost, J. T., & Banaji, M. R. (1994). The role of stereotyping in system-justification and the production of false consciousness. *British Journal of Social Psychology, 33*(1), 1–27.

Kvale, S. (1996). *Interviews: An introduction to qualitative research interviewing*. London, UK: Sage.

Levtov, R. G., Barker, G., & Contreras-Urbina, M. (2014). Pathways to gender-equitable men. Findings from the men and gender equality survey in eight countries. *Men & Masculinities, 17*(5), 1–35.

Libreria Editrice Vaticana. (2016). Comunicado final de la X asamblea general "la dignidad de la procreación humana y las tecnologías reproductivas. Aspectos antropológicos y éticos. Retrieved from http://w2.vatican.va/content/1209eminism/1209/es/apost_exhortations/documents/papa-francesco_esortazione-ap_20160319_amoris-laetitia.html

Maltby, L. E., & Hall, E. L. (2014). Religion and sexism. In A. C. Michalos (Ed.), *Encyclopedia of quality of life and well-being research*. Dordrecht, Netherlands: Springer.

Mannis, V. S. (1999). Single mothers by choice. *Family Relations, 48*(2), 121–128.

Mikołajczak, G., & Pietrzak, J. (2014). Ambivalent sexism and religion: Connected through values. *Sex Roles, 70*(9–10), 387–399.

Minh-ha, T. T. (1986). *Woman, native, other: Writing postcoloniality and feminism*. Bloomington, IN: Indiana University Press.

Mohanty, C. T. (2003). *Feminism without borders: Decolonizing theory, practicing solidarity*. Durham, NC: Duke University Press.

Morris, P. (1996). Community beyond tradition. In P. Heelas, S. Lash, & P. Morris (Eds.), *Detraditionalization: Critical reflections on authority and identity* (pp. 223–249). Cambridge, UK: Blackwell.

Mortar Research. (2023). Women report doing majority of household tasks in relationships. Retrieved from www.starlingbank.com/news/women-report-doing-majority-of-household-tasks-in-relationships/

O'Reilly, A. (2009). *Maternal thinking: Philosophy, politics, practice*. Toronto, Canada: Demeter Press.

Park, L. E., Young, A. F., & Eastwick, P. W. (2015). (Psychological) Distance makes the heart grow fonder: Effects of psychological distance and relative intelligence on men's attraction to women. *Personality and Social Psychology Bulletin, 41*(11), 1459–1473. https://doi.org/10.1177/0146167215599749

Phoenix, A., Woollett, A., & Lloyd, E. (Eds.). (1991). *Motherhood: Meanings, practices, and ideologies* (Vol. 4, Gender and psychology Cross-Cultural Research and Methodology Series). Thousand Oaks, CA: Sage, University of California.

Rawat, P. S. (2014). Patriarchal beliefs, women's empowerment, and general well-being. *Vikalpa: The Journal of Decision Makers, 39*(2), 43–55.

Rhode, D. L. (1997). *Speaking of sex. The denial of gender inequality*. London, UK: Harvard University Press.

Rich, A. (1995). *Of woman born: Motherhood as experience and institution*. New York, NY: Norton & Company.

Roberts, S. O., Gelman, S. A., & Ho, A. K. (2016). So it is, so it shall be: Group regularities license children's prescriptive judgments. *Cognitive Science*, 41(3), 576–600.

Sallam, H. N., & Sallam, N. H. (2016). Religious aspects of assisted reproduction. *Facts, views & vision in ObGyn, 8*(1), 33–48.

Scambor, E., Bergmann, N., Wojnicka, K., Belghiti-Mahut, S., Hearn, J., Holter, Ø., … White, A. (2014). Men and gender equality: European insights. *Men & Masculinities, 17*, 552–577.

Seguino, S. (2011). Help or hindrance? Religion's impact on gender inequality in attitudes and outcomes. *World Development, 39*(8), 1308–1321.

Sidanius, J., & Pratto, F. (1999). *Social dominance: An intergroup theory of social hierarchy and oppression.* New York, NY: Cambridge University Press.

Silverman, D. (2012). *Doing qualitative research: A practical handbook* (4th ed.). London, UK: Sage.

Solomon, S. E., Rothblum, E. D., & Balsam, K. F. (2005). Money, housework, sex, and conflict: Same-sex couples in civil unions, those not in civil unions, and heterosexual married siblings. *Sex Roles, 52*, 561–575.

Stitzlein, S. M. (2008). Private interests, public necessity: Responding to sexism in Christian schools. *Educational Studies. A Journal of the American Educational Studies Association, 43*(1), 45–57.

Tamayo Acosta, J. J. (2011). Otra teología es feminism. Pluralismo religioso, interculturalidad y feminism [Another theology is feminism. Religious pluralism, interculturality and feminism]. Barcelona, Spain: Herder Editorial.

van Egmond, M., Baxter, J., Buchler, S., & Western, M. (2010). A stalled revolution? Gender role attitudes in Australia, 1986–2005. *Journal of Population Research, 27*(3), 147–168.

Witt, S. D. (1997). Parental influence on children's socialization to gender roles. *Adolescence, 32*(126), 253–259.

Yoon, E., Adams, K., Hogge, I., Bruner, J. P., Surya, S., & Bryant, F. B. (2015). Development and validation of the patriarchal beliefs scale. *Journal of Counselling Psychology, 62*(2), 264–279.

Zimmermann, R., & Gygax, P. M. (2016). Women's endorsement of sexist beliefs directed towards the self and towards women in general. In K. Faniko, F. Lorenzi-Cioldi, O. Sarrasin, & E. Mayor (Eds.), *Gender and social hierarchies. Perspectives from social psychology* (pp. 148–158). London, UK: Routledge.

7 Conclusions

This book is grounded in ethnographic research conducted in Spain and the United Kingdom and has offered an examination of the process of deciding to become a "solo" mother using assisted reproductive technology (ART). It provided an analysis of the decision-making process, interactions with healthcare professionals and fertility clinics, the fertility business, public policies regarding access to reproductive technology, managing the balance between work and personal life, childcare, early-childhood education, and children's schooling. The book's objectives revolved around three main themes. First, I analyzed the phenomenon of becoming a solo mother focusing on the use of ART. The second theme explored the role of motherhood and examined how power is exerted through particular social institutions and cultural ideas. In the third theme, I examined solo motherhood and its relationship with reproductive technology as a catalyst for social change.

Feminist perspectives on science encompass more than equity issues, they extend to questions about the ontology, epistemology, and methodology undermining the assertion that social sciences can provide an objective knowledge that is unaffected by the social scientist's personal circumstances. The researcher must be situated inside the same critical framework as the subject of investigation. Traditional ideas and procedures in the social sciences focus solely on the topic of inquiry, as if it exists independently. This social science conceals the manner in which such topics are formed and created inside the tangible and specific social connections where the social scientist actively engages on a daily basis while conducting research. The daily experiences of people inevitably give rise to the "problems" that need theoretical explanations. It serves as the initial foundation for a more comprehensive social science. The factors that influence people's daily experiences are not derived from those experiences themselves but rather from other sources such as the political, legal, economic, technological, and social order. The objective of the social sciences project is to not only reveal the tangible social interactions that shape individuals' realities but also to elucidate the connection between these realities. By drawing upon personal experience and immersing myself in the field which is crucial in anthropological understanding, I have explored two dimensions: my own world and the societal realm that I seek to comprehend. The process of

DOI: 10.4324/9781003269755-8

participant observation involved navigating three distinct modes of engagement with reality: the emotional, the analytical, and the political. By transcending the conventional notion of ethnographic fieldwork as purely intellectual and academic, and recognizing its political and pragmatic implications, a political, ethical, economic, and societal response becomes necessary.

The first chapter provided a comprehensive view of the one-parent family led by women, taking into account the historical, social, political, and religious contexts of both the Franco dictatorship era and the present democracy in Spain. During the Franco dictatorship and the era of National Catholicism, the concept of an ideal family was characterized by the husband's role as the patriarch, mirroring God's position as the head of the church. In line with these ideological parameters, gender differences were viewed as biological and influenced by the celestial order.

Children born out of wedlock were not granted any rights until 1978, when the Spanish Constitution declared that all children were equal under the law, regardless of their parental lineage. In the case of the United Kingdom, the Legitimacy Act 1926 of England and Wales, an illegitimate child could be legitimated by the subsequent marriage of its parents, provided that they were free to marry when the child was born. In 1959, this provision was abolished. Since the Family Law Reform Act of 1969 the rights of an illegitimate child have been broadly similar to those of a legitimate child, though in no case can it succeed to, or transmit a right to, any dignity or title (Camp, 2001).

Thus, when a woman deviated from the social expectation of engaging in sexual activities within marriage, she faced tangible repercussions that were imposed by the government, specifically through its laws and courts, as a matter of public interest. A woman's social standing as a wife or mother was greatly dependent on her sexual propriety. Depriving her of these attributes resulted in her being ostracized from "respectable" society. The church deemed her as the fundamental cause of all deviations from its standards of sexual morality and duly punished her. The child's physical existence served as evidence of a moral wrongdoing, as they were born without a legally recognized father and hence were not allowed to carry their father's last name or inherit his possessions. Therefore examining the legal tradition that considered biological and legal kinship as equivalent reveals that the "natural" family was also governed by legal standards such as marriage, adultery, and illegitimacy. These elements converged to create what Shalev (1989) calls the blood institution, a societal concept that enforced a dual set of rules about sexual reproduction based on patriarchal beliefs about biological sex and the subordination of women. Marriage served, among other purposes, to overcome the question of biological fatherhood by exerting control over women's conduct. The standards around adultery and illegitimacy were primarily punitive measures aimed at women who engaged in sexual activity outside the institution of marriage. Following the development of artificial insemination, there has been a shift in the formation of legal families from biological predetermination to contractual agreements. Thus, ART implies an alternative approach to defining motherhood and parenthood that prioritizes individual autonomy in deciding the outcomes of reproductive activity, rather than relying solely on biological connection. This approach would recognize the constitutional right to privacy for all individuals, regardless of gender, allowing them to have the authority to make autonomous decisions about legal parenthood before conception. In order to adequately defend the interests of the future child and the integrity of the legal family, it is crucial to establish the normative consequences of the reproductive collaboration before the prospective human life begins. The concept of responsibility is a fundamental aspect of this scheme.

Thus, medicalized reproduction affords many new choices, at the same time the authority, to make decisions about those choices has been largely assumed by medical professionals who claim scientific objectivity. In fact, though science as a human endeavor is inherently imperfect, since it rests on observation and comprehension of an environment that is affected by human activity. When human reproduction is the object of inquiry, the nature of the observed process compounds the innate subjectivity of the scientist. Feminist method, as Dorothy Smith (1987) points out, is precisely a critique of objectivity and the aspiration to abstract things from their social context.

Reproductive health is commonly regarded as separate from general healthcare. Instead of being perceived as a medical matter, it is frequently assessed from a moral perspective. When healthcare providers consider reproductive health from a moral point of view, it ultimately becomes a matter of individual decision-making. Consequently, there are doctors, despite their dedication to prioritize the welfare of their patients, who allow their religious beliefs to compromise the standard of care delivered. A contractual framework for establishing the relationship between a mother and a child seems appropriate for the several types of reproductive collaboration made possible by this technology. However, this model is founded on the belief that women are independent individuals, while the history of in vitro fertilization (IVF) shows that medical attitudes still largely reflect the patriarchal notion of women as passive organisms that provide support and are secondary to the value of the human life they conceive.

Doctors may recommend patients to another reproductive clinic based on their religious beliefs, for example, when a woman wishes to become a solo mother with the help of ART and is informed that the clinic only caters to heterosexual couples, or when she seeks embryonic reduction and is advised by her doctor to visit another clinic, despite having assisted her in conceiving through gamete donation, which constitutes discrimination. Commonly, it is women who bear the burden of doctors' religious creeds. The doctors' refusal to administer treatments due to their moral concerns and their capacity to direct patients to other medical centers evokes historical periods when people were denied medical care based on their skin color or ethnic background or legal status. The existence of parliamentary democracies in both countries does not provide a safeguard for women against discrimination in reproductive clinics.

On the other hand, the existing literature on the interaction between the social and biological aspects in societies of the Global North consistently emphasizes the comparison between the traditional nuclear family and newer forms of family. My argument is that this issue is problematic due to two reasons. First, we must challenge the assumption that the biological nuclear family should be used as the standard by which other family forms are measured. Second, by categorizing and generalizing different types of families, we overlook the unique characteristics and variations within each category. The question that arises is why donor-conceived families and adoptive families are consistently compared to biological nuclear families without acknowledging the diverse and intricate nature of each family type. This approach oversimplifies and diminishes the complexity of these families in research studies, erroneously associating genetic relation with kinship or family structure. Some authors repeatedly analyze the children's adaptation in families with donor-conceived children, implying a connection between genetics and the children's welfare. However, they fail to consider research studies that consistently demonstrate that what truly impacts children is not their genetic makeup, the family structure, or the gender of their parents, but rather the presence of caring and secure adults in their homes. According to the findings, the women interviewed considered genetics to be important only in relation to the inheritance of diseases. Furthermore, children's drawings demonstrate the insignificance of genetics since they depict both living and deceased human beings and pets, forming their perception of emotional connections. There is a tendency to overstate the significance of genes and undervalue the influence of the environment, culture, and society; genetic makeup is not a synonym of human identity. Moreover, biological research emphasizes the significance of epigenetics, how environmental factors such as nutrition, stress, and emotions can alter the genes of the donors while in the woman's womb, without altering the fundamental genetic structure. Thus, attributing the issue solely to the child's genes diverts attention from the society where the family is formed. This is especially relevant in societies of the Global North, where the traditional definition of "family" is based on biological nuclear relationships and is influenced by patriarchal, religious, social class, and racialized power dynamics, and thus it must not be taken for granted as a concept. An intersectional methodological perspective acknowledges that families, irrespective of their genetic composition, are shaped by various forms of inequities, for example, singlism, ageism, sexual orientation, social class, ability, racialization, ethnicity, legal status, and religious beliefs. Consequently, the interactions between these different forms of unequal relations may impact the experiences of families and their children.

The ideas of intersectionality are applicable in this scenario since they suggest that social structures are intricate and mutually influence one another. It is necessary to examine families as points where various social structures interact, as sites where power dynamics happen, and as processes that occur inside individuals who are part of culturally embedded groups. The convergence of these perspectives is crucial for analysis, as are diverse reproductive policies, accessible and high-quality childcare facilities that enhance child development, gender, and socio-economic equality. Additionally, I have critiqued the categorization of women who choose to become mothers on their own as "single" or "solo". These phrases perpetuate the dominant perspective of categorizing women based on their absence of a romantic engagement usually with a man. This approach undermines women's ability to make independent decisions and control their own lives. Moreover, the categories "single" and "solo" fail to accurately depict the experiences of the majority of women who were interviewed. These women emphasized the significance of family, friends, social networks, and community groups in their lives.

The book has also provided an overview of the economic landscape around assisted reproduction, a lucrative business valued in the billions. Assisted reproduction clinics, supported by major private investment firms, operate with the expectation of generating substantial profits. These clinics are mostly managed by doctors who may also have financial interests in other connected industries, making them physician-entrepreneurs with overlapping scientific, medical, and entrepreneurial pursuits. ART clinics often exaggerate the "success rates" of treatments and withhold transparent information, making it difficult for patients to have a comprehensive understanding of the overall cost of each treatment from the outset. Most participants in this study were never informed about the potential implications of assisted reproduction treatment, such as unsuccessful efforts, miscarriages, hormone side-effects, or the potential extended duration of attempts required to achieve pregnancy. Furthermore, during this procedure, patients may experience various forms of grief, occasionally accumulating, for which both public and private clinics do not offer psychological assistance. The conflict of interest arising from the intersection of medical and business concerns is evident in the clinics and the experiences of these women. They express dissatisfaction with some clinics, claiming that the clinics may prioritize profit over their well-being. The women are uncertain whether the treatments or tests recommended to them are genuinely necessary or simply aimed at boosting the clinics' financial gains to appease investors. In addition, the national regulatory bodies in both countries have selected members who oversee networks of private clinics specializing in assisted reproduction. These members' economic interests create an ethical dilemma, despite being part of the national commissions associated with the individual ministries of public health, whose primary goal should be to promote the well-being of the general population. Furthermore, public hospitals that provide medical care to patients who pay for their own treatment are mostly funded from general taxation, with additional support from national insurance contributions. Even leading private providers of health services such as Quirónsalud in Spain receives state subsidies through multi-insurance organizations. Public hospitals and private clinics also benefit financially from medical research and medical education funded by taxpayers. Therefore, combining business and medicine can result in unethical practices that betray the confidence of patients. Within a framework of profitable assisted reproductive medicine, physicians may be held responsible to stockholders whose main objective is to generate financial gain. Therefore, medical treatments and counselling that do not have the potential to generate profit, regardless of their effectiveness, are not considered.

Recognizing the complex interplay between mental health, fertility treatment and beyond helps to determine that comprehensive support is paramount. All reproductive clinics must offer all patients the opportunity to talk to a counsellor before they start treatment. Yet, seeing a counsellor is not mandatory, and perinatal mental health services must exist with the aim of pregnant women and new mothers experiencing mental health difficulties to be able to access specialist mental health services everywhere. However, having access to care is only successful if the condition is diagnosed. Unfortunately, in the United Kingdom the National Childbirth Trust's report "The Hidden Half" (2017) found that around half of new mothers' mental health problems do not get identified by a health professional and subsequently treated. Also the report Conecta Perinatal (2022) concludes that there is a high under-diagnosis (between 50% and 75%) of postpartum depression in Europe and Spanish-speaking countries, thus it is necessary to implement strategies that allow its detection and prevention.

Comprehensive mental health assistance must include every phase of an individual's reproductive process, starting from the fertility clinic, continuing through pregnancy, and extending to the postpartum period. By acknowledging and tackling this crucial problem, we have the potential to greatly improve the welfare of mothers and parents, in general, as well as their future offspring. Prioritizing accessible and precise diagnosis, as well as implementing strong support systems, is crucial. In order to secure a better future for families and people seeking fertility treatment, it is vital to adopt a comprehensive approach that integrates medical, psychological, and public policy efforts to help these individuals along their journey. Yet the governments in both countries have entirely failed to implement any measures to safeguard the mental well-being of patients in this field.

Traditionally, women have given birth until reaching the conclusion of their reproductive lifespan. An observable change in recent times is the rising trend of women delaying childbirth till later in life. The decline in the fertility rate in the Global North can be attributed to various significant factors. These include the empowerment of women, their increased access to education and participation in the labor market, improved opportunities for family planning, and the influence of technological, sociocultural, and economic changes. Additionally, the increasing cost of raising children to which the decline of child labor contributed, has also played a role. Moreover, it is crucial to consider the influence of ART and the phenomenon of increased female longevity. Women are increasingly giving birth to their first child at a later age. Discussions in society and the media often revolve around the medical challenges that older women have in carrying a pregnancy and delivering a healthy baby in their late thirties and forties. This often oversimplifies and distorts the scientific understanding of fertility.

The dominant framework of medicalization in the institutionalized treatment of childbirth views the woman giving birth as a passive recipient of interventions rather than an active participant with legal rights. This diminishes their active engagement in the process of pregnancy, labor, and the postpartum period. The legitimacy of obstetric expertise is enhanced by employing a language that presents medical intervention as the most efficient method for reducing mother and baby mortality during childbirth. The institutionalization of reproductive processes replaces women's primary participation in their own pregnancy, childbirth, and postpartum period with the dominance of professional expertise, resulting in an imbalance between obstetric professionals and patients. Moreover, the process of dehumanizing the delivery involves the normalization of violence. Obstetric treatment procedures and tools are applied to women who are seen as just objectified bodies that can be intervened upon. This tacitly denies their human nature and the rights that come with it. All participants in this study are members of the dominant racialized groups in their respective nations, have received a university education, are financially self-sufficient, and have extensively studied and researched their assisted reproduction treatment and preferred method of delivery. Each individual had a sense of empowerment through the utilization of ART, believing that it played a role in providing them with greater authority over their reproductive capabilities and the experience of motherhood. Most participants maintained healthy lifestyles and experienced no complications during their gestation. However, despite these advantages, laboring women were not safeguarded from mistreatment by health staff in public hospitals.

According to the participants interviewed, the obstetric teams did not adhere to the World Health Organization's recommendations that state women with a normal pregnancy and a gestational age of less than 41 weeks should not be induced. Health practitioners should engage in proactive discussions with women in advance if they deem induction of labor to be essential, ensuring that the women comprehend the advantages and potential hazards. Furthermore, it is imperative that women are accompanied by healthcare professionals throughout the entire performance. In addition, the healthcare personnel failed to consider the participants' unanimous preference against undergoing a cesarean section. The medical field is not immune to the ageist and sexist biases that exist in our patriarchal societies. For instance, pregnant women who are over 35 years of age are often labeled as "high risk" and are frequently warned about the potential dangers associated with pregnancy at this age. Additionally, there is a tendency to opt for a cesarean section for women over 35 years of age, even if they have had a healthy and uncomplicated pregnancy. Women who opt to become solo mothers using ART in their late thirties and beyond are making a deliberate choice to assert control over their reproductive decisions and determine the timing of motherhood. These women's life choices elicit heightened moral judgements in society, the media, and the field of reproductive health, subjecting them to punishment for deviating from the societal expectation of conforming to the heterosexual nuclear family model, delaying childbirth beyond the age of 35 years, or asserting their entitlement to receive comprehensive information about medical interventions on their bodies, as well as their right to be treated with compassion, dignity, and respect by healthcare professionals.

On the other hand, the majority of the participants in this study had to pay privately to for ART treatment. A persistent ethical challenge in the field of assisted reproduction refers to the unequal availability of treatments and the potential hindrance of procreative rights due to expensive costs associated with accessing ART. Neither of the two countries where I conducted fieldwork had a comprehensive system of integrated public regulations at the state level that govern and acknowledge solo-parenthood as a legitimate form of family diversity, on par with the heterosexual nuclear family. The lack of a nationwide legislation obstructs the establishment of consistent legal, social, educational, economic, and labor provisions for the rights of solo-parent families, the majority led by women. This reality does not imply that they may all be treated equally without considering and addressing the unique requirements of each family. Incorporating solo parenthood into public policy and social solutions requires abandoning the narrow perspective that associates it exclusively with poverty. The objective is to offer an analysis that can effectively observe, capture, and address the impact of discriminatory situations on women who are both mothers and workers, as well as their children. This is accomplished by considering not just the various aspects of gender but also by examining how the inequities experienced by members of these families intersect with factors such as economy, national origin, gender, abilities, education, culture, and more. The solo-parent family is entirely overlooked in the process of formulating public policies and implementing measures to ensure equality and protection. Hence, addressing this issue demands adopting methodologies that can uncover the complexity of the situation, with the aim of informing public policies and impacting the well-being of these households. Family and personal networks should not bear the burden of resolving everyday challenges trying to balance family and work, and the state should not just engage as a last resort. The legal framework and public policies have the effect of maintaining both the two-parent family model and the obstacles that hinder women from exercising their freedom and responsibility to choose their personal and emotional lives. This system exacerbates the issue of female poverty, particularly among solo-mother homes, as it fails to provide women with adequate protection. An effective policy of equality should address the needs of women who fulfil caregiving and breadwinning roles.

Solo-mother households are not an anomaly. Rather, they must be recognized as a common family form that public policy ought to take into account. By acknowledging solo-motherhood as a component of family diversity, it becomes evident that all types of families share common requirements for emotional and material support. Additionally, specific family circumstances such as being a solo parent, an immigrant, having a large family, being a same-sex or blended family, or being at risk of exclusion, necessitate targeted attention to address their unique needs. Early-education and work–life balance policies must be utilized as essential strategies for fostering a broader perspective and promoting a genuinely collaborative approach that involves and dedicates institutions and society as a whole to transcending the perception of early education and work–life balance as solely the concern of working women. To address the issue of social exclusion, implementing efficient early-education and work–life balance policies can serve as a solution to poverty. These policies allow individuals from working- and middle-class backgrounds to effectively manage their jobs without having to reduce their working hours or quit their jobs to provide care. This creates a safety net for all families. In a recent report, the OECD (2022) emphasized that families have changed at a faster rate than the laws have.

Governments must view well-compensated leave, early-education initiatives, and flexible work arrangements as essential components of co-responsibility with caregiving. These measures ought to be compatible with a socially responsible labor market. Work–life balance is a fundamental right for all people at various stages of their lives. It addresses the needs of different generations and enhances employment conditions, early-education policies, labor well-being, and the productivity of businesses and institutions that implement measures to ensure work–life balance. The demographic phenomenon of population ageing and the issue of gender inequality are urgent and significant difficulties faced by societies in Europe. Addressing these challenges necessitates the implementation of ambitious policies, which include ensuring fair access to assisted reproduction, promoting a healthy work–life balance, and providing high-quality early-childhood education and childcare. These measures would ensure that society as a whole takes shared responsibility for addressing these difficulties. Governments must have a leadership role in delivering comprehensive solutions that coordinate the efforts of many nations grappling with these difficulties, with the aim of attaining a fairer and more sustainable society, along with economic advancement.

Finally this book also examined the motivations behind participants' decision to become solo mothers with the help of ART and explored how their educational choices may disrupt traditional gender socialization practices for their children. Participants described their experience of motherhood as empowering and subversive in relation to the conventional nuclear family. They all expressed criticism towards the outdated masculinity exhibited by their former partners and male acquaintances, while also expressing optimism that future generations will embrace a more nurturing form of masculinity.

Nevertheless, although the literature suggests that non-traditional family structures have an impact due to their members having fewer traditional views on gender compared with their original families, and that factors such as women's higher education, financial independence, professional achievements, and middle-class status can promote more equal attitudes, none of these factors resulted in a significant transformation of the patriarchal ideology among non-feminist participants. These participants hold women responsible for inequality: women's options explain women's disadvantages. They feel uneasy by feminism because it challenges their perception of their own identity and worldview. They perceive social institutions as not playing a role in the creation of inequality and consider affirmative action initiatives to be misguided. They exhibit a lack of awareness on gender issues and refuse to acknowledge gender inequality. Furthermore, non-feminist participants fail to recognize their own personal or political obligation to address this problem. The endorsement of sexist beliefs by women can be attributed to the interpretation of some socially shared norms as inevitable. Johnston (2017) employs the notion of unconscious bias. Unravelling the intricate relationships within the sociocultural network that surrounds these women and from which they have drawn elements to shape their own identity is a challenging endeavor. They refuse to accept feminism and have not developed the necessary awareness to take action and change the current situation. They have the expectation that their children, being the offspring of solo-mother households, understand that both men and women have the ability to perform similar tasks and can achieve social and economic autonomy. However, their decision to enroll their children in Catholic or Anglican schools in Spain and Britain, respectively, reinforces and sustains sexist ideologies. In contrast, half of the participants in this study identify themselves as feminist. They advocate for critical pedagogy in their children's education. They teach their children that their position in society should not be determined by their sex or gender, questioning the government for its deficient public policies and mainstream schools for perpetuating, in numerous instances, patriarchal ideologies. These women do not state that feminism, critical pedagogy, and secular schools are the definitive remedy for social inequity. Nevertheless, they acknowledge that in order to bring about social change, it is imperative that we first undergo personal transformation. For these participants getting involved in feminist and social justice movements with their children contribute to transforming society towards equality and justice appealing to governments to pursue legal and policy change.

References

Camp, A. (2001). Records of illegitimate children. *Family Tree Magazine, 17*(7), 7–9.

Conecta Perinatal. (2022). Mejorar el cuidado de la salud mental perinatal. Alianza hispanohablante por la salud mental perinatal y de la familia. [Improving perinatal mental health care. Spanish-speaking alliance for perinatal and family mental health]. Dr. Pascual Palau (Coord.). Alianza hispanohablante por la salud mental perinatal y de la familia. https://conectaperinatal.com/pdf/ASMI_Memoradum_13sep2022_.pdf

Gaddes, R., Jacobson, Z., Montgomery, S., & Moore, C. (2018). *Conscious and unconscious gender bias*. Insight Policy Research. https://dacowits.defense.gov/Portals/48/Documents/General%20Documents/RFI%20Docs/Dec2018/Insight_RFI%204.pdf?ver=2018-12-08-000555-027

National Childbirth Trust. (2017). *The hidden half bringing postnatal mental illness out of hiding*. NCT United Kingdom. Retrieved from www.nct.org.uk/sites/default/files/2019-04/NCT%20The%20Hidden%20Half_0.pdf

OECD. (2022). Evolving family models in Spain: A new national framework for improved support and protection for families, OECD Publishing, Paris. Retrieved from https://doi.org/10.1787/c27e63ab-en.

Shalev, C. (1989). *Birth power: The case for surrogacy*. Connecticut: Yale University Press.

Smith, D. E. (1987). Women's perspective as a radical critique of sociology. In Sandra Harding (Ed.), *Feminism and methodology* (pp. 84–96). Bloomington: Indiana University Press.

Appendix

Table A.1 List of participants in the United Kingdom and in Spain

Sample in the United Kingdom						
Pseudonym	*Age*	*Color (participants' self-identification)/ Nationality*	*Sexual orientation*	*Profession*	*ART treatment*	*Children*
1. Hannah	43	White Sweden	Pansexual	Musician and executive head-hunter tech industry	Her frozen eggs (at age 37) and non-anonymous sperm donation from the USA	1-year-old son
2. Ruby	48	White UK	Heterosexual	Film TV agent	Double anonymous donation from Spain	2-year-old son
3. Louise	47	White UK	Heterosexual	Director research company	Double donation, egg from her sister and non-anonymous sperm donation from the USA	2-year-old son
4. Mila	38	White France	Heterosexual	Human resources manager	Non-anonymous double donation, egg from the UK; sperm from abroad (she did not want to specify)	3-month-old son
5. Eleanor	37	White UK	Heterosexual	Project manager for high-network travel	Non-anonymous double donation; donor sperm from Denmark and egg from donor in the UK	8-month-old daughter
6. Martine	53	White Belgium	Heterosexual	Physiotherapist	Anonymous sperm donor from the UK and her own eggs	10-year-old son
7. Katya	47	White Ukraine	Heterosexual	Mental health nurse	Anonymous embryo donation in Spain	5-week-old daughter
8. Joyce	48	White UK	Heterosexual	Consultant for a multinational retailer	Non-anonymous sperm donor from the UK and her eggs	9-year-old son
9. Emerald	65	White UK	Heterosexual	Social worker	Anonymous sperm donor from the UK and her eggs	23-year-old son

10. Debbie	60	White South Africa	Heterosexual	Head midwife	Anonymous Jewish sperm donor from the UK and her eggs	17-year-old son
11. Claire	42	White UK	Heterosexual	Senior marketing consultant	Non-anonymous donor sperm from the USA and her eggs	19-month-old daughter
12. Ellen	35	White Ireland	Heterosexual	Patient safety manager	Non-anonymous sperm donor from the UK and her eggs	9-month-old son
13. Susan	54	White UK	Heterosexual	Freelance solicitor, criminal law	Double anonymous donation (sperm and egg) from Spain	10-year-old son
14. Marina	49	White Italy	Bisexual	Yoga and Italian teacher	Double anonymous donation (sperm from Mexican donor in Denmark and egg donor from Greece) at a clinic in Greece	3-year-old son
15. Emily	39	White UK	Heterosexual	Freelance for international NGOs	Non-anonymous sperm donor from Denmark and her own eggs.	2-month-old daughter
16. Nina	39	White Spain	Heterosexual	Manager at UK NGO	Mexican sperm donor from the USA and her own eggs, travelled to Spain for embryo implant	1-month-old daughter
17. Melanie	53	White UK	Heterosexual	Head teacher	Anonymous double donation in Spain	10-year-old daughter
18. Mia	40	White Poland	Heterosexual	Nurse	Non-anonymous sperm donor from Denmark and her own eggs	4-year-old son
19. Isabelle	59	White France	Heterosexual	Accountant	Anonymous double donation in Spain	14-year-old daughter
20. Ella	45	White Ireland	Heterosexual	Software developer	Non-anonymous sperm donor from the UK and her eggs	6-year-old son
21. Chloe	38	White UK	Heterosexual	Human resources manager	Non-anonymous sperm donor from Denmark and her eggs	14-month-old son
22. Olivia	61	White Norway	Heterosexual	Purchasing manager	Anonymous double donation from Spain	16-year-old daughter

(*Continued*)

Table A.1 (Continued)

Sample in the United Kingdom						
Pseudonym	*Age*	*Color (participants' self-identification)/ Nationality*	*Sexual orientation*	*Profession*	*ART treatment*	*Children*
23. Evelyn	46	White UK	Heterosexual	Taxation expert	Non-anonymous sperm donor from the UK and her eggs	8-year-old son
24. Sophie	57	White UK	Heterosexual	Barrister	Non-anonymous sperm donor from the USA and anonymous egg donor from Spain, clinic in Spain	10-year-old daughter
25. Amelia	40	White Spain	Heterosexual	Teacher	Anonymous sperm donor in Spain	2-year-old son
26. Harper	44	White UK	Heterosexual	Associate professor	Non-anonymous sperm donor from the UK and anonymous egg donor from Spain, clinic in Spain	6-month-old daughter
27. Rosie	37	White UK	Heterosexual	Nurse	Non-anonymous donor from the UK and her eggs	1-year-old son
28. Grace	51	White UK	Heterosexual	Analyst IT company	Non-anonymous sperm donor in the UK and her eggs	13-year-old son
29. Alice	43	White UK	Heterosexual	Mathematician	Non-anonymous donor in the USA and her eggs	8-year-old daughter
30. Clara	39	White UK	Heterosexual	Medical doctor	Non-anonymous sperm donor in the UK and her eggs	3-year-old son

Sample in Spain

Pseudonym	*Age*	*Color (participants' self-identification)/ Nationality*	*Sexual orientation*	*Profession*	*ART*	*Children*
1. Gema	43	White Spain	Heterosexual	Social worker	Anonymous sperm donor in Spain and her own eggs	4-year-old daughter
2. Carol	51	White Spain	Heterosexual	Administrative	Anonymous double donation in Spain	5-year-old son
3. Lia	38	White Argentina	Heterosexual	Lecturer	Anonymous sperm donation in Spain and her eggs	3-year-old son
4. Marta	38	White Spain	Heterosexual	Human resources manager	Anonymous sperm donor in Spain and her eggs	10-month-old daughter
5. Raquel	55	White Argentina	Heterosexual	Psychoanalyst	Anonymous double donation in Spain	13-year-old son
6. Carmen	42	White Spain	Heterosexual	Pharmacist	Anonymous double donation in Spain	14-month-old son
7. Vera	47	White Spain	Heterosexual	Freelance, creative advertising company	Anonymous embryo donation, from a woman who used her egg and a sperm donor Spain	7-month-old daughter
8. Eva	48	White Spain	Heterosexual	Translator	Anonymous sperm donor in Spain and her own eggs	2-year-old son
9. Noelia	36	White Spain	Heterosexual	Teacher	Embryo donation from anonymous frozen gametes in Spain	6-month-old daughter
10. Rosa	54	White Spain	Heterosexual	Journalist	Anonymous sperm donation in Spain and her eggs	10-year-old daughter
11. Irene	39	White Spain	Heterosexual	Architect	Anonymous sperm donation in Spain and her eggs	8-month-old son

(*Continued*)

Table A.1 (Continued)

Sample in Spain						
Pseudonym	*Age*	*Color (participants' self-identification)/ Nationality*	*Sexual orientation*	*Profession*	*ART*	*Children*
12. Miriam	56	White Spain	Heterosexual	Biologist	Anonymous double donation in Spain	11-year-old daughter
13. Lidia	54	White Spain	Heterosexual	Solicitor	Anonymous sperm donor in Spain and her eggs	10-year-old son
14. Nerea	49	White Spain	Heterosexual	Sociologist	Anonymous sperm donor in Spain and her eggs	14-year-old daughter
15. Sara	53	White Chile	Heterosexual	Entrepreneur	Anonymous double donation in Spain	12-year-old son
16. María	46	White Spain	Heterosexual	Civil servant	Two anonymous sperm donors in Spain and her eggs	4- and 6-year-old children
17. Julia	54	White Spain	Heterosexual	Secretary	Anonymous double donation in Spain	7-year-old daughter
18. Nuria	39	White Spain	Heterosexual	Economist	Anonymous double donation in Spain	10-month-old son
19. Alicia	57	White Argentina	Heterosexual	Graphic designer	Anonymous sperm donation in Spain	12-year-old daughter
20. Claudia	42	White Spain	Heterosexual	Psychiatrist	Anonymous sperm donation in Spain	2-year-old daughter
21. Mamen	53	White Spain	Heterosexual	Accountant	Anonymous donated embryo implant in Spain	9-year-old son
22. Flor	36	White Spain	Heterosexual	Speech therapist	Anonymous sperm donor in Spain	6-month-old daughter
23. Ainhoa	45	White Spain	Heterosexual	Web developer	Anonymous double donation in Spain	3-year-old daughter

24. Fátima	57	White Spain	Heterosexual	Dentist	Anonymous sperm donor in Spain	12-year-old son
25. Olga	38	White Spain	Heterosexual	Teacher	Anonymous sperm donor in Spain	18-month-old son
26. Alejandra	59	White Spain	Heterosexual	Medical doctor	Anonymous sperm donor in Spain	14-year-old daughter
27. Rocío	41	White Spain	Heterosexual	Medical doctor	Anonymous double donation in Spain	4-year-old son
28. Estela	53	White Spain	Heterosexual	Professor	Anonymous double donation in Spain	9-year-old daughter
29. Matilda	42	White Spain	Heterosexual	Chemist	Anonymous sperm donor in Spain	2-year-old daughter
30. Amparo	36	White Spain	Heterosexual	Teacher	Anonymous sperm donor in Spain	7-month-old son

Source: Author's own data collection.

Index

Made in the USA
Columbia, SC
27 October 2026

781ab74e-dd9e-4147-9987-581bd7d7d189R01